Edited by Elena Hernández-Jiménez

OILY SKIN, ACNE, AND POST-ACNE

IN COSMETIC DERMATOLOGY & SKINCARE PRACTICE

Cosmetics & Medicine
Publishing

Editor:
Elena I. Hernández-Jiménez, *Ph.D.*

Contributors:
Vera I. Albanova, *M.D., Ph.D., Prof.* Dermatologist
Irina Yu. Bragina, *M.D., Ph.D.* Physiotherapist, gerontologist, laser therapist
Natalia G. Kalashnikova, *M.D.* Surgeon, dermatologist, laser therapist
Natalya N. Nikolaeva, *M.D., Ph.D., Associate professor.* Dermatologist, psychologist
Diana S. Urakova, *M.D., Ph.D.* Dermatologist, laser therapist
Alisa A. Sharova, *M.D., Ph.D., Associate professor.* Dermatologist, gerontologist

OILY SKIN, ACNE, AND POST-ACNE
IN THE COSMETIC DERMATOLOGY AND SKINCARE PRACTICE

Many books have been written about acne, but all focus on drug therapy. Unfortunately, the possibilities of modern skincare and aesthetic tools in helping patients with acne are still underestimated. We decided to correct this injustice and created a book in which we present skincare and aesthetic tools, methods, and approaches to preventing and treating this disease. The application of each method is justified in terms of the pathogenesis of acne and is supported by research findings. Describing the events that unfold in the skin after a particular treatment helps in elucidating its clinical possibilities and limitations.

Significant advantages of the book are clear language (although we write about complicated things and use medical and scientific terminology, the information can be understood even by laypeople) and structure (all cause-and-effect connections become apparent, there is a complete understanding of what needs to be done and why).

The book consists of four parts. The first part discusses the clinical signs and stages of acne and distinguishes the acne types amenable to skincare treatments from those that are not.

The second part deals with the diagnosis of acne. It presents recommendations on visual examination and anamnesis collection and discusses the need for clarifying laboratory test results. Much attention is paid to the differential diagnosis of acne with dermatoses like *Malassezia* folliculitis, rosacea, and demodicosis.

The third part presents the factors contributing to the development of acne, explains the pathogenesis of this disease, and outlines the targets to be treated and prevented.

The fourth part is devoted to the practical use of skincare and aesthetic tools and methods at different acne stages — oily skin, non-inflammatory and inflammatory acne, and post-acne. Clinical effects of topical skincare products, injectables, cosmetic devices, and nutraceuticals are discussed.

ISBN 978-1-970196-25-2 (paperback)
ISBN 978-1-970196-00-9 (eBook — Adobe PDF)
ISBN 978-1-970196-24-5 (eBook — EPUB)

FirstEditing

English version is edited and certified by the FirstEditing.Com, Inc. (USA).

Author/Editor

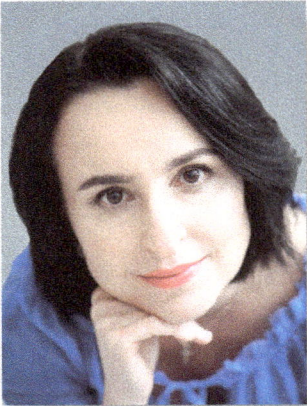

Elena I. Hernández-Jiménez, *Ph.D.*

Biophysicist, scientific journalist

Editor-in-chief of Cosmetics and Medicine Publishing

Chairperson of the Executive Board of the International Society of Applied Corneotherapy (I.A.C.)

Author and co-author of numerous publications in professional magazines, co-author and editor of the book series *Fundamentals of Cosmetic Dermatology & Skincare*, *Cosmetic Dermatology & Skincare Practice*, *Cosmetic Chemistry for Dermatology & Skincare Specialists* and others

Speaker at international conferences, author of training seminars and webinars for professionals in the field of skincare

Professional interests: biology and physiology of the skin, skin permeability, cosmetic chemistry, anti-age medicine, physiotherapy in dermatology and aesthetic medicine, skin analysis and imaging

Table of Contents

PART I

CLINICAL MANIFESTATION

PART II

EXAMINATION & DIAGNOSIS

PART III

ETIOLOGY & PATHOGENESIS

PART IV

SKINCARE AND AESTHETIC METHODS & TREATMENTS

Abbreviations

ACTH	— adrenocorticotropic hormone
AHAs	— alpha hydroxyacids
ALA	— aminolevulinic acid
ATP	— adenosine triphosphate
COCs	— combined oral contraceptives
DHEA-s	— dehydroepiandrosterone sulfate
DHT	— dihydrotestosterone
DNA	— deoxyribonucleic acid
Er:glass	— erbium glass laser
Er:YAG	— erbium-doped yttrium aluminum garnet laser
Er:YSGG	— yttrium scandium gallium garnet laser
FDA	— Food and Drug Administration
FSH	— follicle-stimulating hormone
GCSs	— glucocorticosteroids
HA	— hyaluronic acid
INCI	— International Nomenclature of Cosmetic Ingredients
IR	— infrared light
IPL	— intense pulsed light
KTP	— potassium titanyl phosphate crystal laser
LED	— light emitting diode
LH	— luteinizing hormone
LLLT	— low-level laser (light) therapy
MLA	— methyl aminolevulinic acid
MMP	— matrix metalloproteinase
MSH	— α-melanocyte stimulating hormone
NADH	— nicotinamide adenine dinucleotide hydride
Nd:YAG	— neodymium-doped yttrium aluminum garnet laser
NMF	— natural moisturizing factor
OPCs	— organofluorine compounds
PCA	— pyrrolidone carboxylic acid
PDL	— pulsed dye laser
PDT	— photodynamic therapy

PRP   — platelet-rich plasma
PUFA   — polyunsaturated fatty acid
PTI   — prothrombin index
QS   — Q-switched
RF   — radio frequency
RAR   — retinoic acid receptor
ROS   — reactive oxygen species
RXR   — retinoid X receptor
SPF   — sun protection factor
TCA   — trichloracetic acid
TEWL   — transepidermal water loss
TGF-β   — transforming growth factor beta
TNF-α   — tumor necrosis factor alpha
TS   — testosterone
UV   — ultraviolet light

Introduction

Acne is a problem that, sooner or later, almost all of us face. Some people prefer to ignore this issue, hoping that "it will pass by itself." Sometimes acne does go away, leaving no trace.

But often, things do not unfold so well, and a few non-inflammatory lesions turn into many bright inflammatory lesions that are difficult to treat and can leave a "memory" of a lifetime. So do not let the process take its course; it is better to seek immediate help from a specialist.

It must be said that today's patient has a choice to go to a dermatologist or an aesthetician. The dermatologist has the entire arsenal of registered medications at their disposal, along with the official *Acne Management Guidelines*, which provide a medical treatment scheme.

Aesthetician can utilize a wide range of different cosmetic techniques. Even if they are not included in the *Guidelines*, their benefits can be significant.

In this book, we present **modern cosmetic products, methods, and approaches to the acne prevention and treatment**. For patients and professionals, this is probably the most exciting information, and we will make sure that it is presented clearly. We will not consider drug therapy as it is covered extensively in the *Acne Management Guidelines.*

But first, we will discuss three fundamental aspects that will determine the treatment choice and application.

We start with the **clinical picture** and describe the external signs and forms of acne disease. They are quite variable but also quite characteristic. Acne, in most cases, is tough to confuse with any other condition. However, it is possible and if this happens, treatment will not work and can worsen the patient's condition. Therefore, proper **diagnosis** is one of the critical aspects determining the success of treatment and preventive measures. There is another point — in some forms of acne, aestheticians alone cannot resolve the issue and it is necessary to seek help from other doctors. So, the beautician has to consider the question: "Is this my patient?" If the answer is yes, the beautician proceeds to create an individual treatment program and select specific techniques. For this, understanding the **etiology** and **pathogenesis**, that is the causes and mechanisms of the development of the disease, is necessary.

Part I

Clinical manifestation

1.1. Acne evolution and stages

Acne typically produces external signs that make it easy for a skincare specialist (and everyone else) to recognize them. The different types of acne lesions come together to form an overall picture by which you can determine the severity and the clinical type (**Fig. I-1**).

The acne lesions have different outward manifestations. An **open comedo** is a dark spot visible on lighter skin. A **closed comedo**, although not contrasting in color, is still visible because it is elevated above the skin and has the appearance of a slightly lighter bump. But papules, pustules, nodules, and cysts are distinguished not only by their size and shape but also by their red color, signaling inflammation.

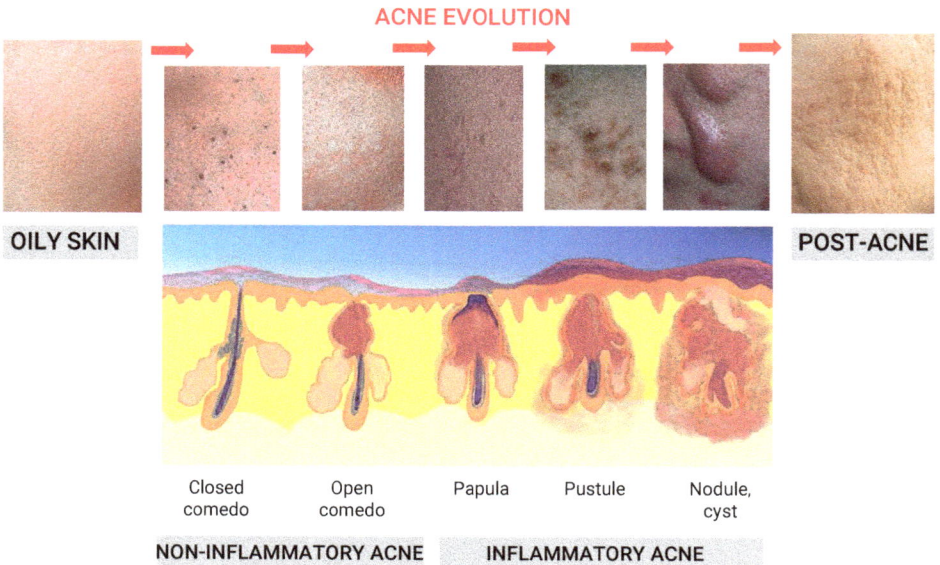

Figure. I-1. Acne manifestation and the stages of acne

An acne patient usually has different types of lesions; together, they form a clinical picture by which to judge the severity of the disease and its clinical type.

We draw attention to an essential practical point: **acne lesions evolve**, i.e., gradually pass from one form to another. Lesions must be considered in dynamics as stages of acne.

It all starts when the sebaceous glands begin to work harder and produce more sebum. Usually, the oily substance secreted by sebaceous glands, sebum, easily pours onto the skin's surface and spreads over it, mixing with the sweat to form the so-called **hydrolipid mantle**. This mantle not only softens the skin. It protects skin from drying out and contacting with external substances, controls the microbiome (a community of microorganisms living on the skin that plays a vital role in its health), and influences the formation of the *stratum corneum* and its barrier structures.

At the beginning of the disease, the outflow of sebum is not impeded; it just forms in greater quantities than usual. Outwardly it is manifested by a characteristic greasy sheen, enlarged pores, and some stickiness. Patients sometimes note that it feels like "there is some heaviness" on the skin.

Over time, sebum production becomes excessive and its physical characteristics change: viscosity increases, its fluidity decreases, it no longer comes out of the pore so quickly and begins to accumulate in it, and finally, the pore is clogged. Not being able to escape to the skin's surface, sebum accumulates in the ducts of the sebaceous glands which become bloated over time. At this stage of development of acne lesions, we see slight bumps on the skin, which can also be felt under fingertips — these are closed comedones (or miliums).

At the skin surface, due to the contact with air, lipid oxidation occurs, and sebum becomes darker. Here, various external substances (particles of pigments in decorative cosmetics, dust particles) are mixed in. The result is a dense plug of dark, almost black color, which clogs the sebaceous duct and is known as **open comedo (blackhead)**.

But sebocytes continue to work. At some point, the wall of the sebaceous gland cannot withstand the pressure and begins to crack. Through these micro-cracks, sebum enters the intercellular space. Usually, it should not be there, so immune cells react to it as a pathogen — an inflammatory reaction begins. We can see this because the skin in the affected area turns red and the white bump turns into a red **papule**.

But the process doesn't stop there. Now, the immune cells penetrate sebaceous glands, forming pus — a mixture of immune cells, bacteria, fragments of sebocytes, sebum, and enzymes. In the center of the papule a whitish patch appears. This is pus, which tells us that the inflammation process has moved into the sebaceous gland, the next stage in the evolution of acne lesions — the **pustule**.

At this stage, the following can happen. The sebaceous gland wall ruptures, and pus ends up inside the skin. It begins to "sprawl" over the skin tissue, forming large, solid, painful lumps under the skin (**nodules**) that can merge to form **cysts**. Very rarely, pus gets into the blood — and sepsis begins. The pathological process involves the epidermis and derma, and the integrity of the basal membrane is disturbed. As a result, after the inflammation is complete, scars, enlarged pores, and most likely post-inflammatory pigmentation will remain in this area. The skin enters the **post-acne** stage — this is not a disease, but an aesthetically unacceptable skin condition, with which the person has to continue to live, sometimes causing irreparable damage to their self-esteem.

What conclusion can we draw? It is obvious. **The earlier the pathological chain is interrupted, the more likely it is that we can stop the process in its early stages.**

Drugs are not necessary in the early stages. What is required are the following measures:

- Periodically clean the pores and remove comedones, so they do not stretch the pores.
- Regularly and properly cleanse the skin of external impurities and remove hyperkeratosis around the mouths of the sebaceous glands so that the pores are not clogged.
- Moisturize the skin to allow the formation of a coating that mimics the normal hydrolipid mantle.

- Gently reduce sebum production activity with topical retinol and salicylic acid preparations.
- Use special skincare products with a protective effect, as acne-prone skin is sensitive.

This is a recipe for acne prevention, which in many cases will help bring the situation under control in the initial non-inflammatory stages. Still, it needs to be noted that its success rate depends on the clinical type of acne.

1.2. Clinical types of acne not to be treated by aesthetician

Who can count on the help of an aesthetician?
The bad news is that local topical management with skincare products won't work for everyone. The good news is that it will work for most acne patients.

Alas, some types of acne require other specialists who "work" on a systemic level (**Fig. I-2**).

Neonatal acne, also known as *acne neonatorum*, is one of these cases. It is an acneiform eruption that occurs in newborns or infants within the first 4–6 weeks of life, and presents with open and closed comedones on the cheeks, chin and forehead. The pathology is diagnosed in approximately one-third of newborns. The leading cause of neonatal acne is a hormonal crisis. Newborns have high levels of maternal sex hormones in their bodies. In addition, the child does not have a fully formed endocrine system, which cannot cope with its functions. If the pimples run without complications, there will be no trace in a few weeks. But an inflammatory process begins if an infection gets into an infant's skin. Pimples transform into pustules, which form pus. In this case, medication therapy is necessary.

Acne against the background of **metabolic disorders** also require specialist treatment. People with an elevated body mass index often experience acne lesions resulting from a severe hormonal illness. A consultation with an endocrinologist is necessary here.

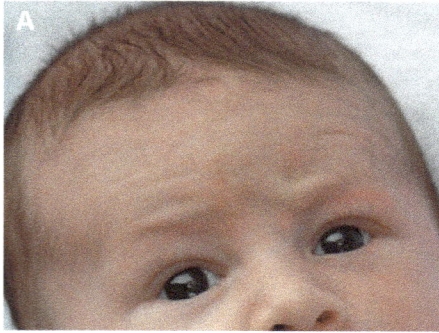

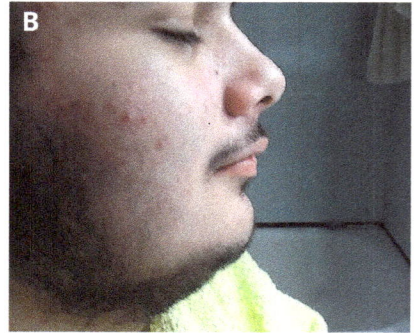

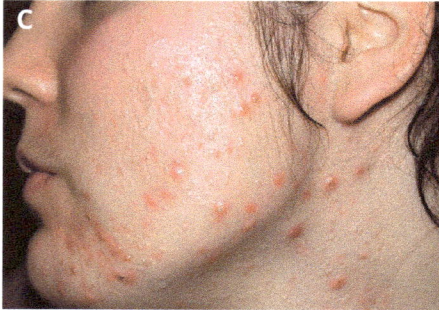

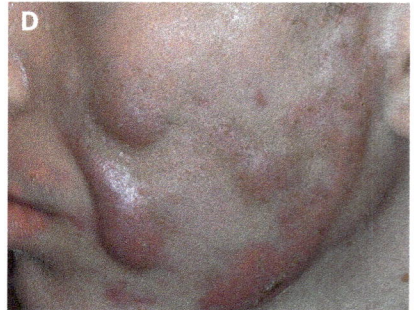

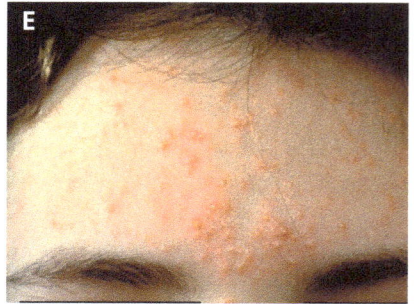

Figure I-2. Routine skincare is ineffective for: A — neonatal acne (Image by Wikipedia); B — metabolic syndrome (Image by Wikipedia); C — hyperandrogenism (Image by Dermatoweb.net); D — conglobate acne (Image by Healthline.com); E — steroid acne (Image by Huidziekten.nl)

Acne appears in **hyperandrogenism** against the background of an increase in the level of androgens in the body. In such situations, you should consult an endocrinologist and a gynecologist.

Long-term use of certain medications can provoke acne (**drug-induced acne**). For example, acne occurs while taking glucocorti-costeroids (GCSs), anabolic steroids, androgens, thyroxine, barbi-turates, cyclosporine a and even some vitamins (B_1, B_2, B_6, B_{12}, D_2).

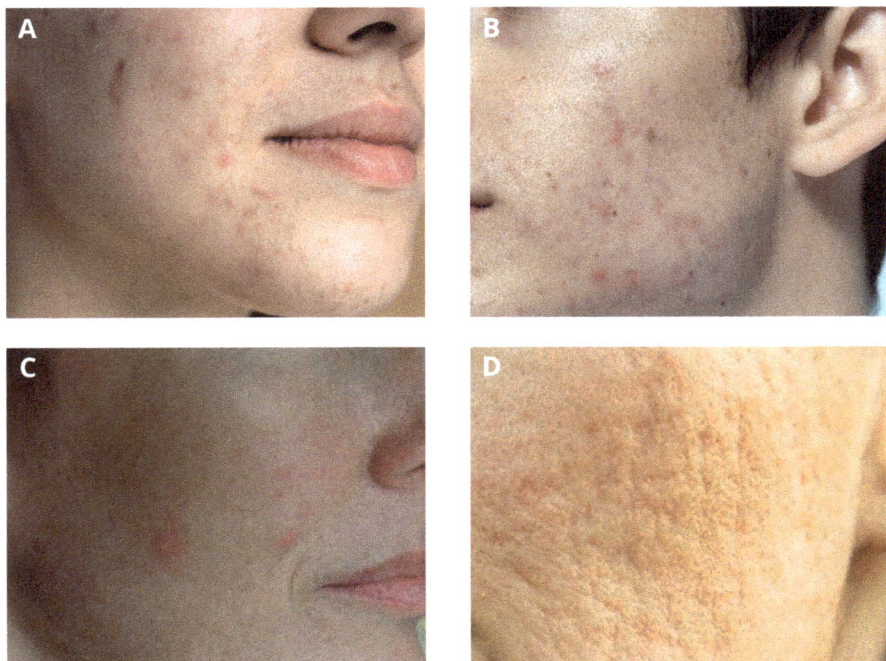

Figure I-3. Aesthetician's patients: clinical types of acne in which aesthetic skincare is effective: A, B — *acne vulgaris* (Image by Freepik); C — *acne tarda*; D — post-acne

These medications can aggravate existing acne. And no matter what the beautician does, as long as the patient takes these drugs, he treatment will not be successful.

Severe inflammatory types with nodules and cysts (**conglobate acne, indurative acne**) are also not amenable to cosmetic treatment. Here we need medication therapy and even surgery.

But some of these patients can be helped by an aesthetician (**Fig. I-3**). The most common types of acne, teenagers' *acne vulgaris* and late-onset *acne tarda*, are amenable to cosmetic treatments. Although these types are also the result of an imbalance in the body's regulatory systems, working with the skin on a local level will yield results.

An aesthetician can help patients with **post-acne**. In fact, for treating post-acne syndrome (scars, enlarged pores, post-inflammatory pigmentation), the same methods and approaches as those used to reduce age-related skin changes and signs of photoaging (wrinkles, age spots, uneven tone) are effective.

Résumé

Acne is a chronic disease of the sebaceous glands, resulting from a disturbance of the mechanisms that regulate their activity. The pathological condition has a characteristic clinical picture, develops gradually, and lasts a long time — until the regulation is restored. In most cases, you can control the course of the disease and try not to let it evolve. Whether this will be achieved with cosmetics or drugs depends on the acne severity and type.

Diagnostics will help us to decide on the treatment strategy and will help determine its likely outcomes.

Part II

Examination & diagnosis

The diagnosis of acne is usually uncomplicated and based on the clinical picture. Nonetheless, diagnosis is necessary to determine the exact cause of acne and decide whether treatment by other specialists is required.

Another factor that cannot be discounted is that acne can resemble other types of inflammatory dermatosis. But the pathophysiological mechanisms of its appearance will be different, and it should be treated differently. All this needs to be understood before treatment is started.

1.1. General examination and anamnesis gathering

1.1.1. What to look for besides the lesions

First, we should look for signs of systemic severe **hormonal abnormalities**, such as hyperandrogenism and metabolic syndrome (see **Fig. I-2**).

Hyperandrogenism, an excess of male sex hormones, can occur in both women and men. In women, the most prominent signs of hyperandrogenism are hirsutism, baryphonia (a low, rough voice), a male physique, and irregular menstruation. Men with hyperandrogenism may have enlarged mammary glands. In both cases, acne is not uncommon. Hormonal correction improves the skin's condition, but a dermatologist or beautician alone cannot help such patients.

Metabolic disorders (disorders of lipid metabolism, carbohydrate metabolism) will manifest in excess weight and metabolic syndrome. Such patients often have acne that is resistant to dermatological and aesthetic treatment. The lesions go away as the overall metabolism is restored.

1.1.2. What to ask the patient at the first visit

Ask if the patient's immediate family members (parents, grandparents) have had acne. Acne is a **genetically predetermined disease**; if there is a family history of acne, the risk of its emergence increases. However, genetic predisposition is only a probability, not a 100% certainty. Under favorable circumstances, you may not have the disease, or it may not be as severe.

But some factors can provoke and aggravate the disease. They include everything that can disturb the delicate balance of regulatory mechanisms and start a pathological process such as:

- Acute or prolonged psychological stress
- Improper nutrition
- Certain medications (see Part I, section 1.2) and contraceptives
- Heavy physical activity

In a conversation with the patient, it is necessary to identify the presence of these factors and further try to level them out.

1.2. Laboratory tests

There are cases in clinical practice when a patient is not examined at all or, on the contrary, is reviewed so thoroughly that a logical question arises — **why?** It is always necessary to understand why a comprehensive analysis is done and what will change in the treatment if a deviation from the norm is detected. In what cases and for what purpose are acne tests prescribed? Let's name three reasons:

1. To identify factors involved in the pathogenesis and influencing the course of the disease
2. To prescribe systemic therapy and physiotherapy
3. To monitor response to certain medications

1.2.1. Sex hormone test

Examining sex hormones is highly relevant because impaired production or reception of sex hormones is a critical factor in acne pathogenesis. In adolescence, a surge in the production of sex hormones is a physiological phenomenon, so most patients of this age do not require an examination since the level of hormones is within the physiological norm. In adolescents, only apparent abnormalities in the development and functions of the genitals are grounds for examination. In other age groups, acne can be associated with severe health problems, mainly endocrine and oncological diseases. The indications for examination are outlined below.

In children:
- Symptoms of hyperandrogenism: early sexual and physical development, early body odor, early prepubertal acne

In women:
- Symptoms of hyperandrogenism: late acne (first appearing after age 25), sudden acne with a pronounced exacerbation before menstruation, stress-induced acne resistant to therapy (including systemic retinoids)
- Symptoms of androgen-dependent dermatopathy: seborrhea, hirsutism, diffuse androgenic alopecia
- Signs of virilization: low voice (baryphonia), male physique, hirsutism, enlarged clitoris
- Symptoms of polycystic ovaries: irregular menstruation, anovulation, infertility
- Symptoms of metabolic syndrome: insulin resistance, hypertriglyceridemia, rapid weight gain, increased blood pressure
- Symptoms of hypoandrogenism: painful intercourse (dyspareunia), decreased libido, diffuse androgenetic alopecia, rare and sparse menstruation or cessation, unexplained weight gain, apathy, sleepiness, and depression

In men:
- Symptoms of hyperandrogenism: enlargement of the external genitalia, excessive and early appearance of body hair, and rapid musculature development
- Symptoms of metabolic syndrome: insulin resistance, hypertriglyceridemia, rapid weight gain, increased blood pressure

It is recommended that **only a few of the essential hormones** be included in the initial examination:

- Testosterone (TS), total and free
- Androstenedione
- Dehydroepiandrosterone sulfate (DHEA-s)
- Follicle-stimulating hormone (FSH)
- Luteinizing hormone (LH)

Examination for sex hormones is recommended:

- At least one month after discontinuation of hormonal contraception and hormonal therapy
- On an empty stomach
- At rest (not after stress, running, etc.)

One day before drawing blood, refraining from alcohol, smoking, sexual contact, and physical activity is desirable. Men may take a hormone test on any day subject to these conditions. In women, the timing will depend on the cycle phase: progesterone and estradiol on days 21–22 (luteal phase) and the remaining hormones on days 3–5 (follicular phase). The beginning of the cycle is considered to coincide with the 1st day of menstruation.

1.2.2. Microbiological test

Growth of the anaerobic Gram-positive bacteria *Cutibacterium acnes* (*C. acnes*; former name — *Propionibacterium acnes*, *P. acnes*) in the sebaceous follicles is a significant component of the pathogenesis of acne. However, their presence is rarely detected in the skin scrapings and through pustule contents analysis.

The fact is that a culture of *C. acnes* can only be obtained on special media, usually not used in bacterial testing, unless specifically requested. Other skin inhabitants, most often aerobic microorganisms, such as the saprophytic epidermal *Staphylococcus epidermidis*, always grow more readily on conventional media. Its sensitivity to antibiotics is recorded in the tests. Thus, for *C. acnes*, it is advisable to perform a bacterial culture in suspected Gram-negative folliculitis (usually *Klebsiella* or *Serratia* Gram-negative anaerobes are found) or *Staphylococcus aureus* infection.

1.2.3. Before planning systemic retinoid therapy

This examination includes blood biochemistry and pregnancy tests.

Biochemical blood test

The biochemical blood test includes evaluation of the following parameters: total protein, cholesterol, high and low-density lipoproteins, triglycerides, urea, creatinine, alanine aminotransferase, aspartate aminotransferase, total and direct bilirubin. Blood for the test can be drawn at any time of day. Still, many factors affecting even healthy people will force them to resort to repeated analyses when some of the indicators fluctuate or deviate from the normative values. Therefore, it is better to follow the **rules for taking a biochemical blood test**:

- Fasting 8–12 hours prior to the test
- Consume light dinner the evening before, after which you can only drink pure water
- Avoid increased physical activity the day before the test
- Do not take a hot bath at night
- Do not take pills in the morning
- Do not exercise
- Do not be nervous

Pregnancy test

Commercial tests with a sensitivity of at least 25 mIU/ml are used to determine pregnancy. The first test is performed after the decision on the need for retinoid therapy, and the second and third tests are performed respectively on one of the first three days of the menstrual cycle and when commencing treatment (these days may coincide). If menstruation is irregular, the test is performed three weeks after unprotected sexual intercourse, and retinoid treatment is initiated only after one month of effective contraception.

1.2.4. Before prescription of combined oral contraceptives (COCs)

The examination protocol includes:
- Measurement of blood pressure
- Heart rate
- Body mass index (no more than 30 kg/m^2)
- Biochemical blood tests (for indicators, see Part II, section 1.2.3)
- Gynecological examination (mammary glands, cytological examination of cervical mucus)
- Pregnancy test (must be negative)
- Coagulogram indicators: activated partial thromboplastin time (APTT) prothrombin index (PTI), fibrinogen, thrombin time (TT)

The study of blood clotting parameters is best performed on an empty stomach or 8 hours after a meal, excluding alcohol consumption for one day and smoking for 2–3 hours. Patient should be advised to drink a glass of water before taking the blood.

1.2.5. Before physiotherapy

The examination includes:
- Clinical blood test
- Urine test
- Electrocardiogram (for patients over 40 years old)
- Consultations with a therapist and a gynecologist

1.2.6. Laboratory monitoring during retinoid therapy

Control biochemical analysis is prescribed 2–4 weeks after the beginning of therapy. Thereafter, it should be repeated every three months if there are no deviations.

1.3. Differential diagnostics

Unfortunately, diagnostic errors may occur, so the prescribed treatment will be ineffective. Moreover, the skin condition may worsen, especially if the diagnosis is made hastily and based solely on the clinical picture. Performing **differential diagnostics** as early as possible is necessary to avoid such situations.

The three skin diseases that can be confused with acne are:
- *Malassezia* folliculitis
- Demodicosis
- Rosacea (papulopustular type)

1.3.1. *Malassezia* folliculitis

As the name implies, this disease is caused by the fungus *Malassezia* (*Pityrosporum*), which lives on the surface of our skin. *Malassezia* (*Pityrosporum*) folliculitis can easily be confused with the papulopustular type of acne because its clinical picture is dominated by papules and pustules (**Fig. II-1**).

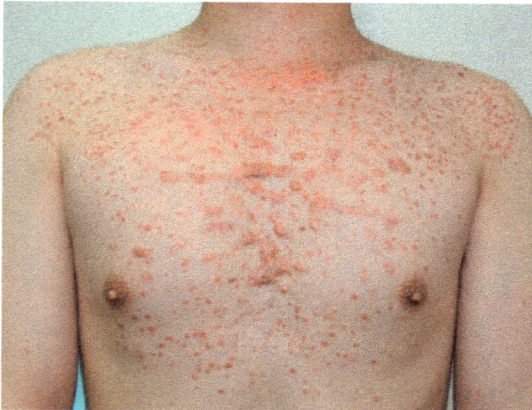

- It is caused by the *Malassezia* fungus
- Men have the disease more often than women
- Anamnesis often reveals systemic and/or topical use of GCSs, antibiotics (often tetracyclines), and immunosuppressants, prescribed for concomitant diseases (diabetes mellitus, Itsenko–Cushing's syndrome)

Figure II-1. Papulopustular lesions in Malassezia folliculitis (Image by Wikipedia)

When collecting anamnesis, systemic and/or local use of GCSs, antibiotics (especially tetracyclines), immunosuppressants, diabetes mellitus, and Itsenko–Cushing's syndrome are often revealed. But this is not the main criterion for the diagnosis.

Table II-1 presents the differences between acne and *Malassezia* folliculitis, which relate to the localization and nature of the lesions and the disease development. There are quite a few, increasing the chances of a correct differential diagnosis. In complicated cases, you can always turn to laboratory tests to help identify the causative agent.

Some concomitant forms, such as acne complicated by *Malassezia* folliculitis, may occur against the background of prolonged use of tetracycline group antibiotics and topical antibiotics.

Accession to fungal infection is an undesirable side effect of antibiotic therapy. This is another argument in favor or prescribing antibiotics only in extreme cases rather than as a preventive measure.

Table II-1. *Malassezia* folliculitis vs. acne

MALASSEZIA FOLLICULITIS	ACNE
Chest, back, less often face	Often face only
Periphery of face and chin	Middle part of the face
Monomorphic lesions (papules, pustules)	Polymorphic lesions, comedones
Itching, burning sensation	No subjective sensations
Rapid improvement due to antifungal therapy	No effect from antifungal therapy
No effect from antibacterial therapy	Antibacterial therapy is effective
Frequently repeated antibiotic therapy in anamnesis	Antibiotic therapy in anamnesis is not obligatory
Deterioration in summer months	No
Deterioration in warm, humid environments, during and after physical activity	No

1.3.2. Demodicosis

Demodicosis is another dermatosis that can be confused with acne. It is caused by a mite of the genus Demodex, which lives in the ducts of the sebaceous glands and feeds on sebum. Mites are active at night, at high temperatures (30–40 °C) and humidity, so itching bothers patients mostly at night, and exacerbations occur in the summer, especially among frequent visitors to the bath and sauna, as well as workers in hot shops and kitchens.

There are two types of demodicosis (**Fig. II-2**). *Demodex* folliculitis is characterized by erythematous spots, papules with scales, and pustules on the face and scalp. Dry, flaky, rough skin is noted. The lesion may be unilateral. In the papulopustular type of demodicosis, the lesions tend to be symmetrical and are located mainly around the eyes and mouth.

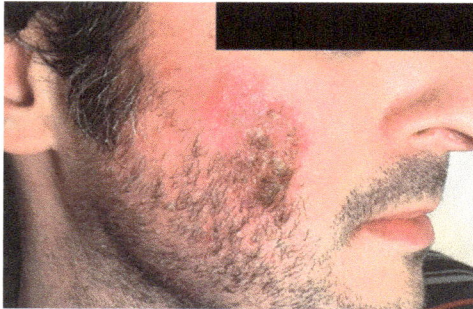

***Demodex* folliculitis:**
- Erythematous spots, follicular papules with scales on the surface, pustules on the face and scalp
- Dry, flaky, rough skin
- The lesion may be unilateral

(Image by Casas M.N. et al., 2020)

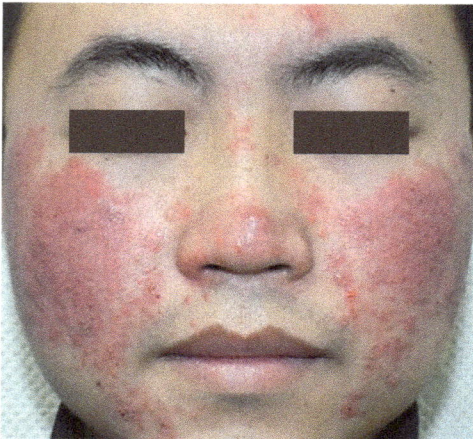

Demodicosis (papulopustular type):
- Lesions are predominantly perioral and periorbital
- Dense erythematous areas, often symmetrical

(Image by Ran Yuping et al., Wikipedia)

Figure II-2. Lesions in demodicosis

Late onset of the disease (after the age of 30), lack of association with hormonal influences, and characteristic subjective sensations will help to suspect demodicosis (**Table II-2**).

Table II-2. Demodicosis vs. acne

DEMODICOSIS	ACNE (PAPULOPUSTULAR TYPE)
Onset in adulthood (30–60 years old)	Onset in adolescence
Worsening with age	Improvement with age
No association with hormonal effects	Connection to sex hormones
No comedones	Open and closed comedones
Only the face is affected	Lesions on the chest and back
Lesions around the mouth and eyes	No tendency to occur around the mouth and eyes
Frequent lesions on scalp	No lesions on scalp
May have unilateral presentation (*Demodex* folliculitis)	Always symmetrically distributed
Itching, sensation of touching fuzz, usually at night	No subjective sensations
Worsening in summer and heat	Usually improves in summer
No scarring	Often post-acne scars
Often blepharitis, conjunctival hyperemia	No ocular involvement

1.3.3. Rosacea

Another condition often confused with acne is rosacea (papulopustular type), in which inflammatory papules and pustules appear on the skin (**Fig. II-3**). Microcirculatory disorders cause rosacea. It is unrelated to the sebaceous glands and can occur at any level of sebum production. Persistent dilation of the capillaries in the skin results in congestion in the skin tissue. Various cells in the affected area begin to malfunction. With time, the structure of the skin changes: the barrier of the *stratum corneum* is violated and becomes more permeable to foreign agents, the activity of immune cells increases, inflammatory

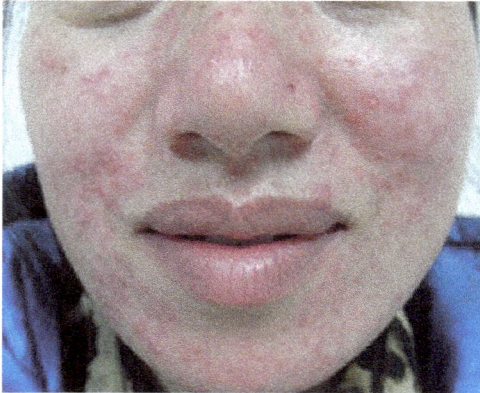

- Rosacea is caused by an imbalance in the microcirculation of the skin
- Characterized by (1) erythema (flares at the beginning of the disease and persistent redness after that) and (2) telangiectasias
- Responds to vasodilatory triggers: insolation, extreme temperatures, spicy and hot food, alcohol, stress and excitement, local irritants, and vasodilating medications

Figure II-3. Papulopustular type of rosacea (Zhou M. et al., 2016)

processes begin, persistent intercellular edema develops, and puffiness occurs.

Careful anamnesis and physical examination will help rule out rosacea because the emergence and initial manifestations of this dermatosis are not characteristic of acne (**Table II-3**).

Table II-3. Rosacea *vs.* acne

ROSACEA (PAPULOPUSTULAR TYPE)	ACNE
Onset during adulthood (30–60 years)	Onset during puberty
Worsening with age	Improvement with age
No connection to hormonal effects	Connection to sex hormones
No comedones	Open and closed comedones
Only the face is affected	Lesions on the chest and back
Erythema flare	No erythema flare
Erythema centrofacialis, telangiectasias	No erythema or telangiectasia
Exacerbation with insolation	Improvement with insolation
No scarring	Frequent post-acne scarring
Often blepharitis, conjunctival hyperemia	No ocular involvement

Detailed information about skincare products and treatment for rosacea-affected skin is available in the *Rosacea and Couprerosis in Cosmetic Dermatology & Skincare Practice* book.

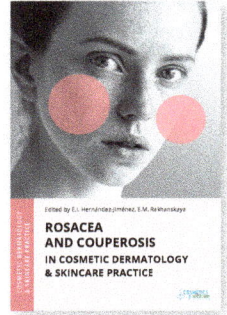

Edited by E.I. Hernández Jiménez, S.M. Rakhmanskaya

ROSACEA AND COUPEROSIS
IN COSMETIC DERMATOLOGY & SKINCARE PRACTICE

Résumé

We did a visual examination, took a medical history, and ensured that this was "our patient" and that we could help. To do this, we have many different tools at our disposal — cosmetics, skincare devices, injectables, and nutraceuticals.

What to choose? Understanding the etiology and pathogenesis of acne will help us answer this question.

Part III

Etiology & pathogenesis

Why do some people have acne and others do not?

Why do some people get sick for a long time, severely and with consequences, despite all the efforts taken, while the process proceeds imperceptibly for others?

What factors can provoke and aggravate this disease?

What happens in the skin affected by acne?

Let's consider each of these questions in turn.

1.1. Oily skin-related dermatoses

The microbiome of oily skin is always altered. This is understandable because the hydrolipid mantle is the primary habitat for microorganisms living on the skin.

Environmental changes inevitably affect the microbiome, disrupting normal skin's natural microbiological equilibrium. The situation becomes even more complicated when the immune system is weakened and/or the patient is taking antibiotics. Under such conditions, the growth of some microorganisms may be activated, while that of others will be suppressed. This is bad for the skin because its health depends on the state of the microbiome.

A consequence of dysbiosis is a skin disease. For example, in persons with oily skin, the **activation of *C. acnes* will result in acne** (Dréno B. et al., 2018), yeast-like fungus Malassezia — seborrheic dermatitis or Malassezia folliculitis (Saunte D.M.L. et al., 2020). Sometimes, these microorganisms behave aggressively, and the patient will have "acne and seborrheic dermatitis" or "acne and *Malassezia* folliculitis." The risk of **demodicosis** is also higher in oily skin because the *Demodex* mite feeds on sebum (Aktaş Karabay E., Aksu Çerman A., 2020).

1.2. Seborrhea

Seborrhea is a commonly used synonym for **seborrheic dermatitis**, a skin disorder characterized by inflammatory scaling lesions in seborrheic areas of the body.

Not everybody develops seborrhea, only those with a genetic predisposition. Seborrhea has three peaks of activity:
1. In the first three months of life
2. During puberty
3. In people aged 40–60 years

1.2.1. Causes

Seborrhea most often occurs during puberty, against the background of hormonal restructuring and imbalance between male and female hormones. Seborrhea with onset during puberty is called **physiological seborrhea**. Physiological seborrhea usually resolves at the end of puberty.

Typically, seborrhea is caused by hormonal malfunctions associated with the increased production of androgens. As a result, the stimulation of androgen-sensitive sebaceous glands increases, and they begin to produce an excess of sebum. In women, seborrhea manifestations are associated with androgen/progesterone imbalance (an increase of androgens and a decrease of progesterone and estrogens). In men, the cause is an increase in androgen levels and acceleration of androgen metabolism, possibly due to hereditary factors and the presence of androgen-producing tumors (e.g., a testicular tumor).

Increased skin oiliness is often observed in HIV-infected patients, as well as individuals suffering from Parkinson's disease and Itsenko–Cushing's syndrome. Psychiatric disorders (schizophrenia, manic-depressive psychosis), epilepsy, biotin hypovitaminosis, and long-term use of certain medications (e.g., testosterone, progesterone, anabolic steroids, GCSs) may also be risk factors for seborrhea.

1.2.2. Signs and symptoms

There are two clinical variants of seborrhea: **oily** and **dry**. It is possible to encounter a mixed type: in this case, some areas of the skin are affected by dry seborrhea, while others exhibit from manifestations of oily seborrhea.

Oily seborrhea

The clinical signs of oily seborrhea are oily shine, stickiness, and enlarged pores on the face, which can be clogged (comedones). With a prolonged course, the skin takes on a grayish hue (looks "dirty").

This condition occurs more often in young women and is usually accompanied by vasomotor disorders. During puberty, sebum production increases unevenly in the different seborrheic areas: increased sebum production is particularly prominent on the face and scalp. A large amount of monounsaturated oleic acid appears in the sebum composition, which liquefies the sebum.

Oily seborrhea with few, non-inflamed blackheads on the nose and cheeks is so common among young people that it is almost normal (physiological seborrhea).

Dry seborrhea

Compared with the oily type, dry seborrhea is associated with lower sebum production, and the sebum is more viscous and not as evenly distributed on the skin. Sebaceous pores may not be very enlarged, but corneocyte keratinization and desquamation are impaired. This is manifested by visible flaking (dandruff on the scalp), which can be accompanied by inflammation and itching.

Dry seborrhea shows all the signs of dry skin with compromised barrier function, although the barrier is also severely compromised in oily seborrhea.

1.3. Acne

Acne is a chronic inflammatory disease manifested by open or closed comedones and inflammatory lesions such as papules, pustules, or nodules. As has already been stated, the background for the development of acne is oily skin, a condition associated with excessive sebum production and a change in lipid composition.

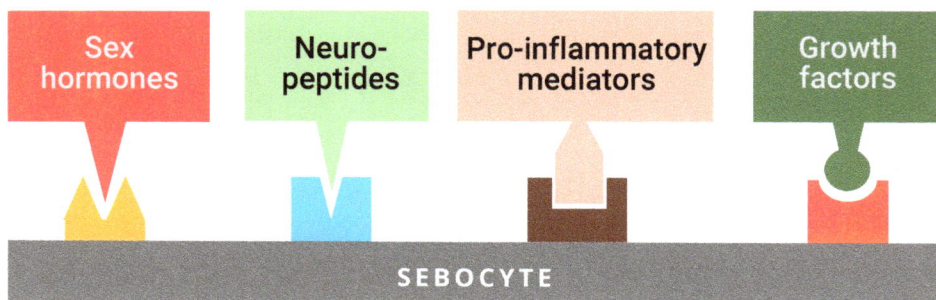

Figure III-1. Sebocytes have receptors to a wide range of signal molecules

What makes the sebaceous glands work so actively? Signals to the sebocytes that trigger the synthesis of sebum lipids. Sebocytes have receptors for many regulatory substances, not just sex hormones (**Fig. III-1**). Some are neuropeptides and inflammatory mediators (Clayton R.W. et al., 2020). These substances are involved in general and local regulation, "acting" on behalf of other regulatory systems — the nervous and immune systems. Some growth factors — besides controlling skin regeneration — also influence sebocyte activity. One or more of these systems may malfunction at once. We aim to determine the "weak link" and understand where the main therapeutic "blow" should be directed. But it's not that simple.

The fact is that regulatory systems always work in tandem (Contassot E. et al., 2012). Today we are increasingly talking about neuro-immunoendocrine regulation, emphasizing the interconnection of all these systems. Accordingly, if there is an imbalance in one of them, the work of the others will also be affected (Tan J.K.L. et al., 2018). We can isolate the primary disruption — where it all came from. But we must understand that it is a chain reaction, and "misalignment" at one site will invariably lead to disruption in other places.

This also applies to sebocytes. There is a leading trigger (often a hormonal link), but the nervous and immune regulatory mechanisms are also affected. Therefore, acne is a multifactorial disease; its pathogenesis involves several trigger factors and several pathological chains simultaneously.

Let's take a closer look at them.

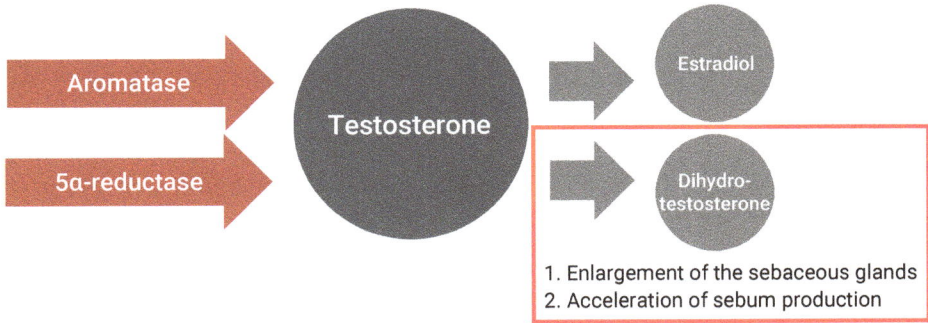

Figure III-2. Hormonal factor in acne development: imbalance of sex hormones in favor of male hormones

1.3.1. Causes

Hormonal factor

In most cases, the primary factor in acne is hormonal (**Fig. III-2**) (Arora M.K. et al., 2011; Barrault C. et al., 2015).

A strong trigger for sebocytes is dihydrotestosterone (DHT). It is formed from testosterone by the enzyme 5α-reductase. It is this enzyme (not testosterone) that triggers seborrhea.

Testosterone also serves as a raw material for synthesizing female sex hormones — estrogen — this happens under the action of the aromatase enzyme. Estrogens, unlike DHT, reduce the activity of the sebaceous glands. 5α-reductase and aromatase compete for a substrate in the form of testosterone.

Under what conditions do DHT levels increase? One reason is that the amount of the precursor substrate in the body may increase and testosterone production becomes excessive. This can be a physiological story (remember the three peaks of seborrhea manifestation!) or a consequence of endocrine pathology (Sekhon A.K. et al., 2020). When blood testosterone levels rise, DHT levels increase, resulting in increased sebaceous gland activity and seborrhea.

Another reason is that 5α-reductase is too active and competes more successfully with aromatase for testosterone. This also happens, for example, in hyperandrogenism in women and it has to do with genetics.

Psychogenic factor

It is well-known that stress increases the skin oiliness and exacerbates acne. This happens because sebocytes have receptors to biologically active substances involved in the development of stress at the systemic (body) and local (skin) levels (Pondeljak N., Lugović-Mihić L., 2020).

Thus, sebocytes are sensitive to acetylcholine, the primary neurotransmitter in the cholinergic nervous system that is directly involved in the development of the stress response in the body. Acetylcholine directly stimulates sebum production (Borrel V. et al., 2019).

Sebocytes are also sensitive to some stress hormones, such as adrenocorticotropic hormone. Here, too, the interaction can be direct.

Still, to a greater extent, the connection between the nervous and immune systems is mediated. The stress reaction (i.e., the body's response to an external hazardous stimulus) is triggered in the brain (in the central nervous system) but is realized via hormones: this is the so-called hypothalamic–pituitary–adrenal axis. We will not go into details but will point out that, under psychological stress, there is a sharp change in the hormonal background, and this can affect (and affects!) both sebocytes (increased sebum production) and immunocytes (increased inflammation).

The bottom line is that patients with seborrhea and acne experience an exacerbation in their condition when stressed. Therefore, any measures that help them achieve mental balance (psychotherapy, relaxation procedures, yoga, etc.) positively affect the skin.

To some extent, the psychogenic factor can also be attributed to intrinsic peculiarities because we have different levels of mental stability that are genetically fixed.

Immune factor

Immune performance in patients with acne differs from that of a healthy person (Wang D. et al., 2020). A reflection of this disparity is the change in acne patients' skin and the gut microbiome. Therefore, probiotics are indicated for such patients: they help to restore the microbiome and improve the immune system function.

The state and functioning of the immune system are also primarily related to genetics.

A condition called **neurogenic inflammation** is an example of a complex neuroimmune factor because both nerve and immune cells are involved. It starts due to the irritation of the skin receptors, for example, by chemical irritants, when there is a change in pH or sudden temperature fluctuations. Free nerve endings in the skin respond by releasing inflammatory mediators, which attract immune cells to the area, triggering an immune response (i.e., inflammation), and expand capillaries, providing blood flow (erythema occurs). Inflammatory mediators include substance P and histamine. Besides, in the process of inflammation, immune cells release free radicals, which, on the one hand, neutralize the pathogen (if there is one) and, on the other hand, support inflammation.

Notably, sebocytes also have receptors for substance P and histamine. They perceive these molecules as activating signals. Therefore, the skin's response to stimuli will increase sebum production. Accordingly, **irritation and trauma to the skin should be avoided because inflammation will only increase the already high sebum production**.

Biochemical factor

The clinical picture reflects abnormalities in many intra- and extracellular biochemical processes in the skin, including the following:

- Metabolic reactions, during which the synthesis of sebum lipids takes place. Therefore, acne-prone skin is characterized by the increased synthetic activity of sebaceous glands.
- Production of mediators and signaling molecules, such as pro-inflammatory mediators, immune cell chemoattractants, and reactive oxygen species (ROS), often make acne-prone skin inflamed and hypersensitive.
- Changes in the expression of proteins involved in keratinization (such as filaggrin and involucrin) and *stratum corneum* enzymes (responsible for assembling the lipid barrier at the border of the granular layer and its destruction in the upper layers). This explains hyperkeratosis: the *stratum corneum* thickens, but as its internal organization is disturbed, it begins to perform the barrier function poorly, cannot retain water, and lets foreign substances pass more easily.

In acne-prone skin, the composition of surface lipids — intercellular lipids (which form the lipid barrier in the *stratum corneum*) and those included in the sebaceous production — is altered (Zhou M. et al., 2018, 2020; Esler W.P. et al., 2019). In general, the linoleate content is inversely proportional to the level of sebum production: the more sebum, the lower the concentration of linoleic acid in it.

As for the lipid barrier within the *stratum corneum*, o-acyl ceramides contain the greatest amount of linoleate among all other lipid fractions. In acne, the linoleate content of acyl ceramides is significantly reduced. In acyl ceramide deficiency, sebocytes have increased sensitivity to inflammatory mediators and other substances involved in the pathogenesis of acne (e.g., free fatty acids). In addition, acne is accompanied by a change in the ratio of saturated, monounsaturated, and polyunsaturated fatty acids in the epidermal lipid metabolism.

Linoleic acid deficiency leads to skin alkalinization (surface pH of the acne-prone skin increases on average to 5.8–6.0) and an increase in the permeability of the follicle epithelium, disrupting its barrier function. In addition, a decrease in the linoleic acid concentration contributes to a disturbance in the keratinization processes in the orifice of hair follicles due to the disintegration of corneodesmosomes, which leads to the follicular duct blockage and comedone formation.

Another finding in the skin of acne patients is a decrease in vitamin E and an increase in squalene peroxide levels, indicating their significant role in the sebum lipid oxidation process and the need to strengthen the antioxidant potential of the skin.

Enzymes control all biochemical reactions in our body, and their activity is related to genetic traits.

Anatomical factor

Not all ducts of the sebaceous glands open directly to the skin's surface. Most sebaceous glands are connected to the hair follicle. Humans have lost a continuous hair cover, but even hairless areas have hair follicles producing thin and short fluffy hair.

There is a paradox: sebaceous glands associated with regular hair are small and unilobular, while those associated with downy hair are large and multilobular. The most prominent and branched sebaceous glands are located on the face and upper back. In acne-prone skin, the ducts of sebaceous glands on the face and back are thinner, longer, and more tortuous than in the average person, which makes it difficult for sebum to escape to the skin surface.

The anatomical structure of the sebaceous glands is related to genetics.

Microbiome factor

C. acnes is considered the main factor contributing to the emergence of acne, even though this microorganism is part of the normal human skin microbiome. It belongs to the anaerobes, which means it lives in conditions with little oxygen inside the sebaceous gland filled with a hydrophobic mass.

C. acnes can stimulate sebocytes directly by increasing their synthetic activity (shown in experiments on cell cultures) or can act indirectly.

The primary nutrient substrate for *C. acnes* is glycerol. To obtain it, *C. acnes* enzymatically break down sebum triglycerides, releasing one glycerol molecule and three free fatty acids. Some of these fatty acids interfere with lipid metabolism in keratinocytes, disrupting the keratinization process next to the pilosebaceous duct orifice so that hyperkeratosis develops around it, the pore becomes closed, sebum evacuation is stopped, and sebum accumulates inside the gland. Others (primarily arachidonic) stimulate the production and release of interleukins 6 and 8 by sebocytes, which leads to further intensification of sebum synthesis. Furthermore, the enzyme lipoxygenase can convert arachidonic acid into various immunoreactive substances, activating neutrophils, monocytes, and other cells involved in inflammation.

Accelerated sebum production leads to a predominance of fatty acids synthesized from glucose. At the same time, the relative content of unsaturated fatty acids (linoleic and γ-linolenic), necessary for forming the intercellular lipid barrier of the *stratum corneum*, decreases. Against the background of an improperly formed barrier, the skin's protective function deteriorates, and its permeability increases (Rocha M.A., Bagatin E., 2018). This makes it even easier for bacteria to enter the sebaceous gland, and in addition to *C. acnes*, staphylococci, streptococci, and other agents of purulent infections soon become established there.

Another mechanism of *C. acnes* involvement in the pathogenesis of acne is related to their ability to affect keratinocytes, which react by releasing ROS, such as superoxide anion radicals. When the skin's antioxidant system is imbalanced, ROS released by keratinocytes begin to damage cell membranes, leading to the release of immunoreactive substances that trigger the inflammatory process.

Finally, *C. acnes* can form a bacterial film, a continuous layer of bacteria bound together, rendering them highly resistant to antibiotics and antiseptics. This film disrupts the normal skin exfoliation process and creates further prerequisites for sebaceous gland blockage.

1.3.2. Pathogenesis

The prerequisites for the development of acne are hyperproduction of sebum and a change in its composition.

First, there is more nutrition for *C. acnes*. They take advantage of this and begin to multiply (**Fig. III-3**).

Second, atypical fatty acids appear in the triglycerides of sebum. Obtained from triglycerides, these acids can affect the sebocytes as stimulatory signals. They can also affect keratinocytes, triggering the release of inflammatory mediators and inflammatory responses. Recall that we have already talked about how inflammation itself stimulates sebum production.

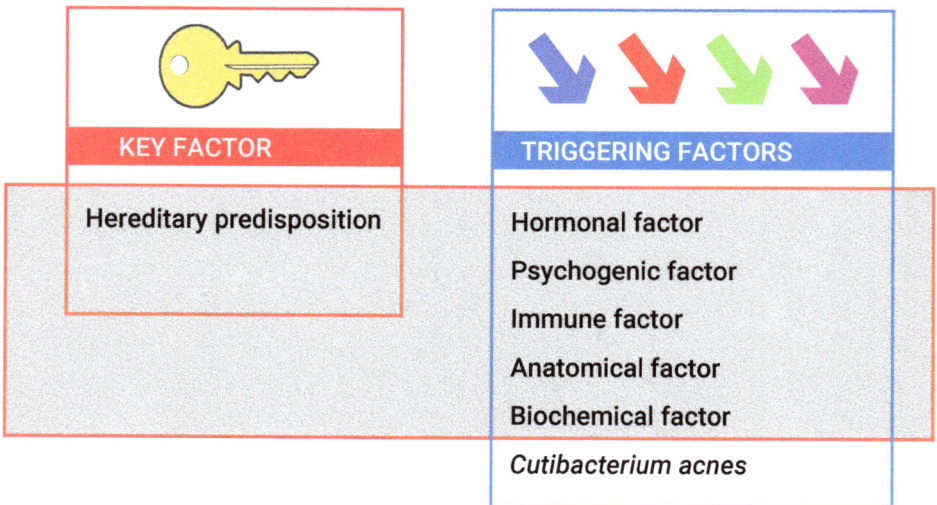

KEY FACTOR	TRIGGERING FACTORS
Hereditary predisposition	Hormonal factor
	Psychogenic factor
	Immune factor
	Anatomical factor
	Biochemical factor
	Cutibacterium acnes

Figure III-3. Acne is a multifactorial disease

This results in a vicious cycle supported by *C. acnes*. But this bacterium is not the one that starts the process! It takes advantage of the favorable opportunity presented by the processes described above.

Yes, *C. acnes* are a factor involved in acne. However, it is not a critical factor but one of the triggers. The key factor in the development of acne is a **genetic predisposition** (Lichtenberger R. et al., 2017; Kanazawa N., 2020), which controls all trigger factors except that related to *Cutibacterium* (**Fig. III-3**). So, the immediate culprit of acne, *C. acnes*, gains strength only on "fertile" soil. This leads to a significant practical conclusion: **antibacterial monotherapy can only temporarily alleviate the condition**. As it will not solve the problem, primary acne therapy should be aimed at strengthening the body (especially its immune system) and normalizing the skin barrier structures.

Résumé

There are four links in the pathogenesis of acne (**Fig. III-4**):
1. Sebaceous gland hypertrophy and increased sebum production
2. Follicular hyperkeratosis
3. *C. acnes* activation
4. Disruption of the microbiome and inflammation

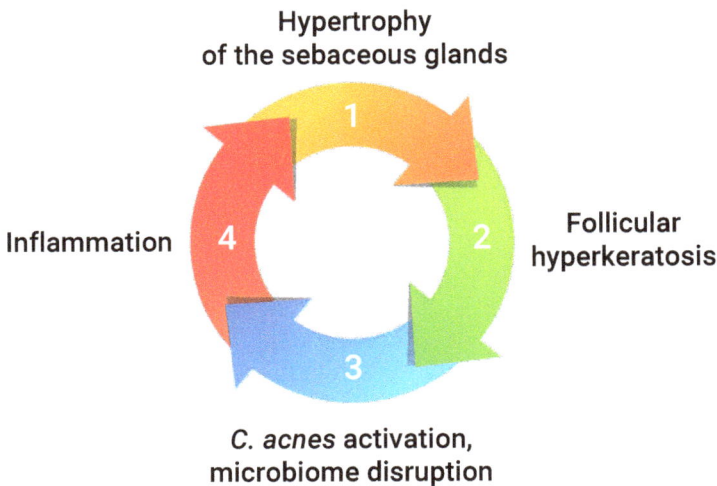

Figure III-4. Dermal "targets" for acne prevention and treatment

These are the dermatological targets that must be treated simultaneously. Today there is a great variety of skincare products for acne prevention and treatment. But there is no universal solution to this problem because acne is a multifactorial disease. It is necessary to fight it simultaneously on different fronts with several provoking factors and focus on restoring several disturbed mechanisms in the body and the skin.

How to choose the right product? How to apply it? These questions are highly important for skincare specialists and their clients or patients. We will answer them in the following chapters in light of the etiology and pathogenesis of the disease.

Part IV

Skincare and aesthetic methods & treatments

Chapter 1
Oily skin

The best acne prevention is to stop it in the earliest stages when the first signs of seborrhea appear. This is entirely feasible with the help of special cosmetic care.

1.1. General recommendations

1.1.1. Identifying the cause and prescribing pathogenetic therapy

It is not difficult to diagnose seborrhea but it is often challenging to determine its cause. In this regard, a skincare therapist or dermatologist often recommends that a patient consults with other physicians. A gynecologist–endocrinologist should examine women because of the risk of high levels of androgens. All patients should visit a gastroenterologist.

The treatment of seborrhea is individual and complex. First, it is necessary to eliminate the cause and provoking factors. For example, if high androgen levels in a female patient are detected, oral contraceptives are sometimes prescribed to normalize the hormonal background.

1.1.2. Special nutrition

The importance of nutrition for optimal health and prevention/management of many conditions is increasingly being recognized. It has long been noticed that acne outbreaks can be provoked by certain foods such as hot spices, fatty foods, and chocolate. This does not mean that these products will cause aggravation in every person with oily skin. But to prevent the emergence of acne, it is still worth limiting their intake.

Conversely, some foods are indicated for people with oily skin. It is recommended (especially during antibiotic therapy) to take probiotic products (Ellis S.R. et al., 2019; Goodarzi A. et al., 2020), i.e., products containing bacteria of normal intestinal microflora — lactobacilli and bifidobacteria. Usually, these are liquid fermented milk products, containing about 10^6 bacterial cells/g.

> **Note!**
> If you suffer from **acne**, you should refrain from dairy products containing sugar and carbohydrate-containing additives (dried fruits, etc.) during antibiotic therapy.
> In **seborrheic dermatitis**, the "milk + simple carbohydrates" combination is ideal for the growth of most fungi, so you must choose plain products without sugar, fruits, or cereals.

By taking certain probiotics, several pathological processes in the skin related to the dysregulation of immunological and/or neuro-sensory mechanisms can be affected and prevented (Yu Y. et al., 2020).

How do probiotics affect the skin while within the gastrointestinal tract? This question has been actively studied in recent years. Much is already known, in particular:

- By restoring and maintaining the digestive function, probiotics enhance health by helping to ensure that nutrients are delivered in the right amounts and on time to all sites of the body, including the skin.
- In the intestinal lumen, probiotics can directly interact with dendritic cells that express dense contact proteins and permeate the monolayer intestinal epithelium. Through the interaction of probiotic bacteria (or their components) with the intestinal epithelium and/or direct interaction with dendritic cells, activation of other immune cells, such as B- and T-lymphocytes, can occur, followed by the release of immune modulators, including cytokines, into the bloodstream. These cytokines, bacterial fractions, and primitive immune cells can be transported through the bloodstream to other organs, including the skin, where they can affect local immune status.

- The ability of specific probiotics to influence the production of regulatory cytokines and growth factors may play a role in rebalancing the skin's immune system and suppressing inflammatory responses.

The results yielded by clinical and laboratory studies are consistent with the speculation that the biological effects of specific probiotic strains "extend beyond" the gastrointestinal tract and manifest in other organs. In particular, *Lactobacillus johnsonii* NCC 533 (strain La1), a representative of the intestinal microflora of healthy adults, is known for its high antipathogenic activity against a wide range of enteropathogenic microorganisms. This strain was found to have another valuable quality: it affects the skin immunity disturbed after ultraviolet (UV) radiation exposure and increases skin resistance to aggressive environmental factors (including UV).

In addition to probiotics, particular nutraceuticals are recommended that contain balanced proportions of active ingredients and have a targeted effect on specific processes in the skin and body. Modern nutraceuticals designed for oily skin can contain substances such as:

- **Magnesium sulfate** — reduces skin sensitivity to neurogenic stress and aggressive exosome factors
- **Pyridoxine** — together with magnesium, helps maintain skin homeostasis and reduces the skin's sensitivity to stress
- **Antioxidants** (such as vitamin C and plant polyphenols) — combat oxidative stress and improve microcirculation
- **Zinc gluconate** r— egulates the sebum production process
- **Omega-3 polyunsaturated fatty acids (PUFA)** complex — strengthens the barrier function, improves local immunity, and reduces inflammation (Rubin M.G. et al., 2008; Mirnezami M., Rahimi H., 2018; Balić A. et al., 2020)

Until recently, nutritionists advised the consumption of brewer's yeast as a source of B vitamins to everyone with oily skin. Today, this prescription is made individually after determining the level of *Candida* activity in the gut. If the fungal microflora activity is elevated, foods containing yeast should be excluded from the diet.

1.1.3. Health promotion

People with seborrhea should spend more time outdoors and enjoy moderate sun exposure. Bathing with sulfuric mineral water has an excellent preventive effect.

Most importantly, it is essential to normalize the psycho-emotional background and restore equilibrium given that a general hormonal failure is a common backdrop for psychological stress, negatively affecting the local regulation of the sebaceous glands.

1.2. Peculiarities of hygiene and skincare

1.2.1. Cleansing

If you have oily skin, it is essential not to cleanse it "deeply" but to do so in a way that does not damage its protective function.

Most people with oily skin perceive it as greasy and dirty, and the urge to cleanse is almost irresistible. Despite all the research that has shown that oily skin has nothing to do with dirt and that gentle cleansers are reasonable even in this case, there is still a great demand for products that create the illusion of "deep" cleansing.

Advertisements for such products claim they go deep into the pores, opening and cleansing them. Their composition may contain ingredients such as denatured alcohol, acetone, essential oils of mint, tea tree, and eucalyptus, surfactants, etc., which cause a feeling of degreasing, cooling (which many people associate with freshness), and dryness. Some of these products cause a tingling and burning sensation, which is perceived by many as a sign that the product is "working." Unfortunately, the skin condition worsens after heavy rubbing with all these products. There are at least a few reasons for this:

- Alcohol, acetone, and surfactants destroy the hydrolipid mantle and lipid barrier. As a result, pathogens (chemical and biological) can penetrate the *stratum corneum* and provoke inflammation.

- Menthol, eucalyptus oil, and other substances with potentially irritating effects irritate sensitive skin nerves, from which neuro-peptides are released, causing inflammation.

Dissolving surface impurities: cleansing agents

If there is increased sebum production, the first thing that comes to mind is to remove the sebum from the skin's surface. However, this is not so easy to do. Even if we rub the skin with alcohol and quickly remove all surface grease, the greasy shine will appear again after half an hour. The fact is that significant amounts of sebum are stored in the acini of the sebaceous gland, where solvents do not penetrate. But the effect of alcohol does not go away. The lipid barrier between the horny scales is destroyed. Recall that the lipid barrier protects the skin from water loss and binds corneocytes to one another, preventing excessive flaking. Therefore, the destruction of *stratum corneum* lipids by degreasing sub-stances (alcohol, acetone, etc.) negatively impacts the skin and causes acne to develop. Frequent skin washing with natural alkaline soap also destroys the lipid layer (but does not empty the sebaceous glands). Therefore, for acne, degreasing lotions and alkaline soaps should never be used. It is recommended to rely solely on cleansers for oily skin (milk, micellar solution) with a pH of about 4.5–5.5 (slightly acidic).

Wash your skin with warm water, not too hot or too cold. At the same time, try not to rub it too hard so as not to traumatize it unnecessarily.

Microcurrent disinfection can be used for delicate skin cleansing, but it should not be done more than once a month, like galvanic disinfection.

Sebum absorption: absorbents

Besides substances inhibiting sebum production, some cosmetic ingredients reduce the skin's oiliness by absorbing fat. The most popu-lar absorbers are:
- Natural minerals in fine powder form: limestone (calcium car-bonate), talc (magnesium metasilicate), zeolite (water-containing aluminosilicate), calcium silicates, clays (kaolin, bentonite), etc.
- Polymers of plant origin: modified starch
- Polymeric granules with a porous surface: allyl methacrylate cross-linked polymers, lauryl methacrylate/glycol dimethacry-late cross-linked polymers, etc.

Absorbents are included in matting products, often as powder. As they vary in absorbency, some matting formulations will work more effectively and for longer than others. Of course, the absorption capacity of even the best fat absorbents is limited, so if your skin produces too much sebum, matting cosmetics will have little effect.

Pore cleansing

To ensure sebum does not accumulate in the sebaceous glands' ducts and subsequently does not turn into comedones, we should conduct periodic cleaning. At home, many people use scrubs and adhesive strips for this purpose, as they stick to the skin, then tear off along with horny flakes. It must be noted that coarse scrubs containing unpolished particles with sharp edges can traumatize the skin, opening an additional gateway to infection. Therefore, preference should be given to soft scrubs with round and soft polyethylene granules instead of particles made of nutshells. As for the strips, although the result of their use may at first seem excellent, with frequent use, the *stratum corneum* becomes thin and has no time to recover, which reduces its protective properties, with all the ensuing consequences in the form of increased sensitivity and irritability. Strips must not be used simultaneously with retinoids, as retinoids make the skin very fragile and easily damaged.

The best way to prevent the formation of comedones is manual cleaning, which is carried out after steaming the face. The periodic performance of such a procedure not only improves the appearance of the skin but also serves to prevent inflammation, which occurs when the walls of the sebaceous glands are blocked.

1.2.2. Restoring the keratinization/desquamation balance and preventing hyperkeratosis

When sebum is excessively produced, it glues horny scales and hinders their desquamation, which negatively affects the keratinization process and creates conditions for hyperkeratosis, one of the factors for fcomedone formation in acne. For prevention, it is recommended to perform a superficial peeling from time to time but in a way that does not cause inflammation.

Exfoliation

Superficial peeling can help remove horny masses and prevent hyperkeratosis.

For the chemical peeling, use formulations with salicylic acid, proteolytic enzymes, and alpha hydroxy acids (AHAs). All these substances normalize the *stratum corneum*'s renewal and prevent sebaceous glands' blockage.

An essential part of the skincare routine for those with oily skin is maintaining a surface pH of 5.5 because oily skin tends to be alkaline. For this purpose, solutions and light emulsions with AHAs are used, which acidify the *stratum corneum*. Depending on the total AHA concentration and the pH, these products can be classified as cosmetics for regular skincare or as chemical peels for periodic intensive treatment (see Part IV, section 2.3.2).

Gas–liquid peeling, ultrasonic peeling, and brushing remove the uppermost horny scales. However, the mechanical treatment, as well as the chemical one, must be very delicate in order not to provoke inflammation. These procedures can also be performed on acne-prone skin but only during remission (see Part IV, section 2.3.1).

Restoring the lipid barrier: physiological lipids

In seborrhea, sebum lipids should generally remain on the surface, penetrate the intercellular spaces, and become embedded in the lipid layers, changing their physicochemical properties and structure. Therefore, physiological lipids in the normal horny layer — ceramides, cholesterol, and free fatty acids — help restore and strengthen the lipid barrier. Application of these substances in skincare products (including on the scalp) increases the skin's resistance to external influences (Takagi Y. et al., 2018). The skin needs adequate supply of essential fatty acids such as linoleic and γ-linolenic acids, as their deficiency can lead to hyperkeratosis in the sebaceous gland ducts and the appearance of comedones. Essential fatty acids can be replenished by taking nutritional supplements (omega-3 PUFA complex) and cosmetic products containing evening primrose oil, borage oil, or blackcurrant oil.

Dense emulsions with fatty acid esters and saturated fat as emollients are not recommended for oily skin because they can provoke comedones (see Part IV, section 2.2.4).

1.2.3. Normalizing the regulation of sebum production

High sebum production results from dysregulation of neuroendo-crine and intracellular sebocyte signaling pathways. In this regard, acting on regulatory mechanisms is one of the key aspects of caring for oily skin.

Restoring the local hormonal regulation

The level of sebum production is under the control of androgens. Sebocytes are considered key androgen homeostasis regulators in the skin due to several androgen-metabolizing enzymes (Fritsch M. et al., 2001). However, it is not testosterone itself but dihydrotestoster-one (DHT), a substance into which testosterone is converted by the enzyme 5α-reductase, that directly affects sebocytes (Inoue T. et al., 2014). It has been experimentally shown that sebocytes begin to proliferate and mature faster when testosterone is added to the culture medium. Maturation for a sebocyte means accumulation of sebum and subsequent destruction with the release of contents in the gland duct (see Part I, chapter 1).

Some oral contraceptives (e.g., Diane-35) and antiandrogens (spironolactone, etc.) reduce skin oiliness. However, hormones are considered medicinal substances and are prohibited in cosmetic products. Instead, the cosmetic industry relies on substances of plant origin — phytoestrogens, which are not human hormones but have hormone-like effects. The action of phytoestrogens on the skin is still understudied, but there is evidence to suggest that some, such as soy isoflavones, may affect sebum production by inhibiting the enzyme 5α-reductase. In addition, isoflavones are effective antioxidants, stimulate collagen synthesis, and strengthen blood vessel walls. Other phytoestrogens can prevent the conversion of inactive testosterone to active DHT in the sebaceous gland. Extracts of soybean, Mexican wild yam, damiana, clover, hops, common nettle, dwarf palm, and other plants are often found in cosmetics for oily skin because of the various phytoestrogens they contain.

It is not really known how effective cosmetic products can be in influencing the skin's hormonal balance, as there are no serious clinical (comparative, large-scale, placebo-controlled, blind) trials available. Nevertheless, clinical experience with such formulations shows that they can improve skin condition (though not for everyone).

For phytoestrogens to realize their properties, it is necessary to ensure their effective delivery to the metabolically active epidermis (Kircik L.H., 2011). Even if we assume that phytoestrogens can reduce skin oiliness, not all cosmetic products containing these substances will act similarly.

Direct regulation of sebocyte activity

The impact on various intracellular signaling pathways involved in sebum synthesis opens many possibilities to modulate sebaceous gland activity. Still, each of the potential regulators needs to be studied in detail.

One of the most studied is **vitamin A** because it has two beneficial effects. First, it stimulates the proliferation and migration of basal keratinocytes, supporting the cellular renewal of the epidermis and controlling keratinization. Second, it directly acts on sebocytes, reducing their activity. Finally, it stimulates the production of the antimicrobial peptide cathelicidin in the dermal adipocytes around the hair follicle, helping the skin fight *C. acnes*.

Please note that the trans-retinoic acid (tretinoin) and 13-*cis*-retinoic acid (isotretinoin) (see Part IV, section 2.1.1) are drugs; in cosmetic products, they are replaced by retinol (the alcoholic form, which is traditionally called vitamin A) and its esters (retinyl palmitate, retinyl acetate, picolinate). The fact is that retinoic acid is the active form of vitamin A that stimulates gene expression by binding directly to the cells' nuclear receptors. Retinol and its esters cannot bind to the nuclear receptors; however, they are natural precursors of retinoic acid — the cells store them and oxidize them to retinoic acid as needed. If retinoic acid is introduced into the body as a part of topical or systemic drugs, cells cannot control its further fate. Since retinoic acid is a highly active compound with a versatile and pronounced effect on the genetic apparatus, we can see the entire spectrum of consequences, both desirable and undesirable. A safer and milder stimulation would be to supply the cells with retinoic acid precursors (retinol or its esters):

in this case, the cells can control the activation process. This approach is known in medicine as **intracrine regulation**. So, the division between medicinal and cosmetic retinoids is relatively straightforward and lies in the ability to interact directly with the receptors: if there is direct interaction, then it is medicine, and if there is no interaction, it is cosmetic.

Sebocytes have nicotinic acetylcholine receptors (n-cholinoreceptors), a subspecies of acetylcholine receptors that provide nerve impulse transmission through synapses and are activated by acetylcholine and nicotine. Experiments show that acetylcholine increases sebum production in a dose-dependent manner while using these receptors' antagonists suppresses it. What does this suggest? First, it tells us how the nervous system influences sebum production. Second, it opens a new and promising way to regulate sebaceous glands by using substances capable of penetrating the sebaceous gland when applied topically and blocking impulse transmission to acetylcholine receptors of sebocytes (Li Z.J. et al., 2013).

Hyaluronic acid (HA) has also been found to have a sebum-regulating effect through CD44-receptors expressed by sebocytes. *In vitro* and *in vivo* experiments have shown that HA has the capacity to reduce sebum lipid synthesis in a dose-dependent manner. This explains the well-known clinical observation that the biorevitalization treatment (intradermal injection of high-molecular-weight native HA) slightly reduces skin oiliness. If this is a positive effect on seborrheic skin, in the case of sebum deficiency, it is undesirable (Jung Y.R. et al., 2017).

1.2.4. Modulation of the skin's immune status

In oily skin, high sensitivity and inflammation indicate an altered immune status. Skincare products restoring local immunity and reducing skin reactivity are meant for oily skin.

Anti-inflammatory measures

Certain substances secreted by the skin's nerve endings, such as substance P, can provoke sebum production. Receptors for histamine (H1-receptors), a mediator of inflammation, have been discovered on sebocytes and the available evidence indicates that histamine activates sebum synthesis (Nettis E., 2005; Pelle E. et al., 2008; Chugunov A., 2011). All this explains the well-known clinical observation: **substances that irritate the skin can provoke sebum production**.

Still, not every skin reacts to irritants through an increase in sebum production as different people may have different sensitivity of sebaceous glands to inflammatory mediators or different threshold levels of irritation which is followed by the release of such substances. Other signaling molecules are also involved in regulating sebum production and sebum size. For example, α-melanocyte stimulating and adrenocorticotropic hormones (MSH and ACTH, respectively) influence sebaceous gland functioning (Zhang L. et al., 2003; Whang S.W. et al., 2011). Since both testosterone and adrenocorticotropic hormone levels increase under stress, it becomes evident that psychological factors play an essential role in increasing skin oiliness.

Dermatologists typically prescribe zinc ointments and powders to treat mainly mild to moderate inflammatory acne. **Zinc** inhibits sebum production and eliminates unpleasant odors (not coincidentally, it is often included in deodorants and preparations for oily skin and hair).

Zinc preparations dry out the skin and reduce sebum production (by acting on 5α-reductase) and inflammation. Zinc inhibits special receptors on the surface of keratinocytes and dendritic cells (Langerhans cells) — so-called Toll-like receptors (Jarrousse V. et al., 2007). These receptors are the "levers" that zinc needs to trigger various biochemical processes at the cellular level, ultimately reducing the severity of inflammatory reactions in the skin.

Zinc salts' solubility is low, making it difficult to include them in formulations. Zinc pyroglutamate, the zinc salt of pyroglutamic acid (syn.: pyrrolidone carboxylic acid, PCA), lacks this disadvantage. PCA belongs to organic acids and plays a vital role in cell maturation and maintenance of the water balance in the *stratum corneum*. It is derived from the amino acid glutamine which is released in large quantities during the hydrolysis of filaggrin. Subsequently, PCA is synthesized from glutamine by the enzymes g-glutamyl-AA synthase and g-glutamyltransferase. In the form of sodium or potassium salt, it is a part of the natural moistening factor and ensures water binding within the *stratum corneum*. Zinc pyroglutamate, therefore, also acts as a moisturizing agent, which is very useful for oily skin. Zinc pyroglutamate (often paired with nicotinamide) can be found in many products for oily and acne-prone skin.

Modulating skin immunity

Some **synthetic peptides** with antibacterial and/or immuno-stimulatory properties can help modulate immune status and soothe the skin. For example, Rigin tetrapeptide (INCI*: Palmitoyl Tetrapeptide-3) is a fragment of immunoglobulin G involved in various physiological processes, including immune functions. Rigin suppresses IL-6 expression by basal keratinocytes, restoring cytokine balance, reducing inflammation, and improving skin condition (like the "hormone of youth" dehydroepiandrosterone, DHEA). The Bodyfensine peptide (INCI: Acetyl Dipeptide-3) also strengthens skin immunity. It stimulates the production of antimicrobial peptides, β-defensins, increasing the skin's resistance to microbiological invasion.

Nicotinamide, a water-soluble form of vitamin B_3, is very useful. Its anti-inflammatory properties are related to its antihistamine effect, its ability to serve as an electron trap, and its inhibitory effect on 3',5'-cyclic-AMP-phosphodiesterase. In addition, nicotinamide directly reduces sebum production in sebocytes.

Brewer's yeast cell wall extract, known for its immunomodulatory properties, can be found in skincare products for oily skin.

Some plant extracts rich in polyphenols and antioxidants (chamomile, aloe, *Centella asiatica*, and many others) have traditionally been popular in cosmetic products designed for oily skin for their soothing, anti-inflammatory properties.

Ozone therapy can improve local immune status due to its pronounced antibacterial and anti-inflammatory effects.

---

* INCI — International Nomenclature of Cosmetic Ingredients.

1.2.5. Normalizing the skin microbiome

Changes in the quantitative and qualitative composition of the hydrolipid mantle and local immunity have severe consequences for the microbial landscape of the skin. Some previously quiet microorganisms begin to multiply actively and aggressively suppress their neighbors.

As a preventive measure, it is recommended to periodically cleanse oily skin with toners containing plant extracts that exhibit antiseptic action (chamomile, calendula, birch, celandine, etc.).

A modern and very promising strategy is using cosmetics that are friendly to skin mycoplasma. Inactivated bacteria (for example, *Bifido*- and *Lactobacilli*) (Knackstedt R. et al., 2020), substances that improve the growth of certain microorganisms, film-forming compounds that enhance adhesion of bacterial cells, etc. can be used as active ingredients in such formulations. An essential factor of probiotic cosmetics is the ability to maintain the pH level of the skin surface.

With **physiological seborrhea**, the best prevention of dermatoses is proper and regular care and compliance with general recommendations.

With **secondary seborrhea**, medicinal treatment is directed at the underlying disease and the elimination of its cause(s). It is not prescribed by a dermatologist but by the appropriate physician. If seborrhea has progressed into chronic dermatosis, however, drugs prescribed by a dermatologist become the centerpiece of treatment. Treatment mustn't override special cosmetic care and general recommendations.

1.2.6. Moisturizing

Patients with seborrhea often complain of dry skin (visible flaking and increased irritability, potentially accompanied by a feeling of tightness). In these cases, an assessment of the skin's functional parameters shows that the *stratum corneum*'s hydration is almost always reduced due to increased sebum production. This can be present at the onset of seborrhea, which is an important signal that the skin's barrier function is at risk. If you do nothing to support it, you will soon see an increase in the **transepidermal water loss (TEWL)** index, which reflects increased water evaporation through the *stratum corneum* and a decrease in the skin's barrier properties.

Why does this happen? The fact is that seborrhea not only causes sebum production, but its lipid composition also changes. The components of sebum begin to seep through the intercellular spaces of the *stratum corneum* and become embedded in its intercellular lipid layers. As a result, the lipid profile of the upper layers of the *stratum corneum* can be significantly changed with the deterioration of barrier properties (Kircik L.H., 2014).

In this case, along with the skincare products regulating sebum production, moisturizing oil-free gels and natural oils rich in unsaturated fatty acids should be prescribed.

In the case of dry skin with increased sebum production, the application order of moisturizers is as follows:
1. Physiological lipids to restore the lipid barrier
2. Gel-based "wet compress" (if necessary) to relieve the symptoms of dryness

1.2.7. Protection

When talking about protection, it is necessary to remember that oily skin is characterized by increased sensitivity so that it can react to any external aggression (UV, pollutants, sudden temperature changes, low humidity, wind, etc.).

There is no specificity among the functionally active ingredients in protective cosmetic products designed for oily skin. The main difference is in the base substances, which should provide even coverage and not cause discomfort. In this regard, preference is given to lightweight emulsions based on silicone oils and hygroscopic polymers.

Résumé

All of this leads to practical conclusions universally applicable to oily skin.

1. Do not irritate the skin. Since neuropeptides released from sensitive skin nerves and histamine released from keratinocytes increase inflammation and stimulate sebum production, all irritants will contribute to the deterioration of acne-affected skin.
2. Do not traumatize the *stratum corneum*. Products that destroy the lipid layer of the epidermis not only open the skin to new bacteria but also allergens and toxins.
3. Don't rely solely on antimicrobials. No matter how brilliant your victory over germs is, it won't last as long as your skin produces excess sebum.
4. Take good care of your immune system. It's essential to keep your digestive system functioning properly, eat a healthy diet, and improve your overall health.

Proper skincare, starting at the first signs of increased sebaceous gland activity, can help prevent the development of acne. In some cases, these measures may not be enough, and acne lesions will still appear. The specifics of dealing with skin with acne symptoms will be discussed in the next chapter.

Chapter 2
Acne-prone skin

The general recommendations for taking care of oily skin are also suitable for acne-prone skin. We should remember that acne is a disease, and preventive measures alone may not be enough. In this case of inflammation, drug therapy may be required. There are specific points when dealing with acne-prone skin which will be discussed in this chapter.

2.1. Drug therapy

The standard dermatological practice for treating acne is prescribing systemic antibiotics with topical retinoids. If this therapy is unsuccessful, the prescription of systemic retinoids and, in severe cases, even the involvement of systemic glucocorticosteroids is considered.

When the clinical picture is dominated by high oiliness and comedones, papules and pustules are absent or isolated, topical retinoids (Retasol, retinoid ointment 0.05% and 0.1%, gel and cream Differin, Klenzit) and salicylic acid are prescribed along with skincare products for oily skin.

If papulopustular lesions are predominantly papular, topical antibiotics (Dalacin gel, Klindovit, Zerkalin solution, levomycetin), retinoids, benzoyl peroxide (Basiron AC gel 2.5% and 5%), and antiseptics (salicylic alcohol, resorcinol) are prescribed.

Severe types of acne require systemic treatment with retinoids (Roaccutane, Sotret, Accutane, retinol palmitate). If there are contraindications, other drugs are used — antibiotics (doxycycline, Unidox Solutab, Minolexin, Wilpafen), zinc-containing formulations (Zincteral, Zinkit), nicotinamide, etc. All clinical types of acne are treated externally, preferably with a combination of different drugs.

While these drugs are prescribed by a dermatologist, other physicians (endocrinologists, gynecologists, andrologists) are responsible for prescribing medicines to correct a patient's hormonal profile.

2.1.1. Retinoids

All living cells in our body need vitamin A. Receptors for its active forms (retinoic acid isomers) are located in the nuclei. Once bound, they trigger the expression of genes that control cell division and maturation (**Fig. IV-2-1**).

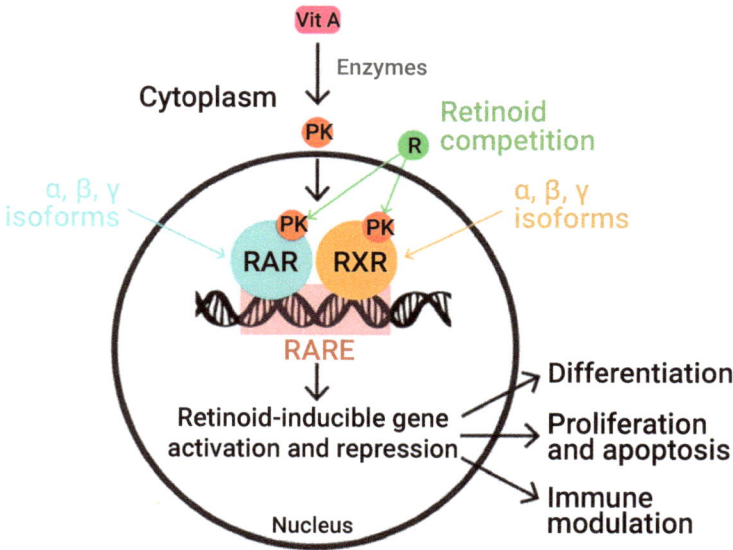

Figure IV-2-1. Retinoid mechanism of action (adapted from Balak D.M.W., 2018)

There are several types of retinoid receptors: RAR (retinoic acid receptors) and RXR (retinoid X receptors), each having three subgroups: α, β, and γ. RAR-γ is expressed predominantly in epidermal cells, RAR-β in dermal fibroblasts, and RAR-α in embryonic skin cells. The activated receptor binds to a short DNA sequence near the promoter of genes that play an essential role in cell proliferation and differentiation. Such binding affects the expression of the corresponding genes, most often leading to the activation and, in some cases, suppression of their expression. The presence of nuclear receptors and similarities in the molecular mechanisms of activation gives scientists the grounds to put retinol on par with steroid and thyroid hormones since their action is also mediated through nuclear receptors. Different types of topical retinoids bind selectively to specific subsets of nuclear receptors and, therefore, have different effects. For example, RAR-γ agonists stimulate the expression of genes involved in barrier defense and epidermal hyperproliferation, while RAR-α agonists inhibit retinoid-sensitive genes.

Therefore, actively dividing cells, which include sebocytes and basal keratinocytes in the skin, are susceptible to retinoids. This explains the clinical effects of retinoids on the skin, a decrease in sebum production, and thinning of the *stratum corneum*.

The skin microbiome also recovers under the influence of retinoids. In 2018, the Journal of Investigative Dermatology published a study exploring the relationship among dermal microbial species, the severity of clinical acne, and tretinoin therapy (McCoy W.H. et al., 2018). Retinoid treatment resulted in a microflora observed in healthy skin. The total number of *C. acnes* decreased, while that of *Staphylococcus* spp. first increased and then fell. The growth of microorganisms such as *Rothia*, *Flavobacterium*, *Enterobacter*, and *Micrococcus* was observed as the disease reached remission. According to the authors, these microorganisms prevented the reproduction of *C. acnes* after the end of treatment.

This is positive news regarding the pathogenesis of seborrhea and acne, but there is a flipside — the barrier properties deteriorate, and skin sensitivity increases dramatically. Patients with a long history of topical medicinal retinoid use have dry, irritated skin with a weak *stratum corneum*. Taking systemic retinoids is fraught with unpleasant consequences associated with flaky and dry skin and mucous membranes, increased skin sensitivity to sunlight, headaches, depression, and digestive disorders (including hepatitis). In addition, retinoids are teratogenic substances, so they are contraindicated for pregnant and lactating women. Other highly unpleasant side effects of taking systemic retinoids (isotretinoin in particular) described in the medical literature include impaired vision (especially during twilight), dry eyes, corneal inflammation, and increased sensitivity to contact lenses.

The retinoids currently used in dermatology (**Table IV-2-1**) are selective agonists of RAR-β and RAR-γ receptors. These are the 1st (retinol, retinal, tretinoin, isotretinoin) and 3rd generation (adapalene, tazarotene) retinoids. The 2nd generation retinoids include etretinate and acitretin, but are not used in acne treatment.

At the end of 2019, the first representative of the 4th generation of retinoids, trifarotene (developed by Galderma), registered under the trade name Aklief, received approval by the U.S. Food and Drug Administration (FDA). Unlike its predecessors, it binds only to RAR-γ, the skin's most common retinoic acid receptor type.

Table IV-2-1. Retinoid drugs prescribed for acne

SUBSTANCE	ORIGIN	DRUGS
Trans-retinoic acid (tretinoin)	Natural active form of vitamin A, 1st generation retinoid	Topical: Tretinoin, Retin-A, Avita, etc.
13-*cis*-retinoic acid (isotretinoin)	Natural active form of vitamin A, 1st generation retinoid	Oral: Roaccutane, Acnecutane, Sotret Topical: Rotasol, retinoid ointment
Adapalene	3rd generation synthetic retinoid	Topical: Differin, Klenzit
Tazarotene	3rd generation synthetic retinoid, derived from β-carotene	Topical: Tazorac
Trifarotene	4th generation synthetic retinoid	Topical: Aclif

The first publications about the new retinoid appeared in 2018 in the British Journal of Dermatology (Balak D.M.W., 2018). According to that study, tripharotene has almost all the therapeutic properties of classical retinoids (anti-inflammatory, comedolytic, and depigmenting) but causes fewer unpleasant side effects such as irritation, flaking, etc., due to its selective binding to RAR-γ (see **Fig. IV-2-1**). In addition, trifarotene has an exciting metabolism. According to the manufacturer, it is stable in human keratinocytes for 24 hours but is almost immediately degraded by hepatocytes, which limits the risks of its systemic effects. Therefore, it can be used on large areas of the skin, which is one of the main advantages of the drug. Presence of extensive acne lesions is the main indication for its use: the FDA has approved the use of Aclif for treating acne on the face and the body (chest, back, and shoulders). The FDA approval is based on the successful results of two Phase III clinical trials involving 2,420 patients which demonstrated that Aclif significantly reduces the number and severity of inflammatory acne lesions on the face (after two weeks) and on the back, shoulders, and chest (after four weeks). The most frequent side effects (incidence

>1%) included irritation, itching, and increased photosensitivity (with the possibility of burns) at the application site. However, the number of such events was low compared to that associated with Aclif's predecessors. Therefore, trifarotene may be helpful for extensive acne lesions and patients with sensitive skin.

2.1.2. Antibiotics

We can assume that an antibiotic agent capable of destroying the microbial content of the sebaceous gland can completely clear the skin of inflammatory lesions. To speed up the process, local antibacterial and anti-inflammatory agents can be prescribed, so that the remaining comedones can be opened, and the gland ducts can be cleaned out. Later, excessive sebum production can be suppressed with retinoids, preventing the development of hyperkeratosis. Such a strategy looks quite logical and reasonable but only at first glance. Although it can achieve a temporary victory over acne, this may soon be followed by a crushing defeat.

Antibiotics often produce rapid improvement, but with their prolonged use, problems begin to emerge. First, against the background of antibiotic therapy, the growth of *C. acnes* and other representatives of the bacterial microflora is suppressed. As a result, fungal microflora may activate, and acne will be joined by seborrheic dermatitis or *Malassezia* folliculitis. Second, antibiotic therapy also negatively affects the intestinal microflora. Since our microbiome is inextricably linked to the immune system, the body's overall immunity eventually declines. As the body's resistance decreases, it becomes easier for germs to get revenge. This explains the exacerbation of acne following a temporary retreat after antibiotic therapy. The problem is usually more pronounced than before treatment and is accompanied by more profound and profuse skin lesions, including the accession of seborrheic dermatitis.

Since many patients wander from physician to physician in search of a cure, and many dermatologists start treatment with antibiotics, you may end up with a severe acne complicated by gut dysbiosis, immune disorders, and the appearance of microbial strains resistant to a wide range of antibiotics.

Undoubtedly, there are cases when antibiotics are necessary, as the prolonged existence of inflammatory lesions (especially deep-seated ones) can lead to irreversible changes in the skin with the formation of fistulas and scars. Still, the prescription of antibiotics should be made very cautiously. Antibiotics can only be a step in acne therapy; the sooner you get past it, the better.

Topical antibiotics can be prescribed alone or in combination with systemic drugs. They are used to treat inflamed areas of the skin. The benefit of topical medications is the absence of systemic side effects. The most common **disadvantages** include:

- Probability of relapse after discontinuation of treatment
- Suppression of skin immunity
- Ability to cause allergic reactions (redness and swelling, scaling, itching of the skin in the treatment area)

Topical drug formulations (**Table IV-2-2**) are mainly produced with antibiotics having a bacteriostatic effect. The primary forms are ointments, gels, creams, lotions, and solutions. Topical antibiotics are applied either across the entire surface of inflamed skin or are dotted on isolated lesions. Combined drugs for topical application that contain, in addition to antibiotics, other active substances act in complex, so they are highly effective.

Antibiotics in tablets and capsules have a more pronounced and sustained therapeutic effect but can cause dysbacteriosis and other adverse reactions from various body systems. **Orally-administrated antibiotics for acne are prescribed if:**

- Inflammation affects large areas
- Infiltrative and cystic types of acne prevail
- Therapy with topical medications does not have a pronounced therapeutic effect

Drugs of the following **pharmacological groups** represent systemic antibiotics for acne therapy:

- Penicillins (Flemoxin Solutab)
- Lincosamides (Lincomycin, Clindamycin)
- Tetracyclines (Doxycycline, Tetracycline)
- Macrolides (Erythromycin)

Table IV-2-2. Topical antibiotics used in acne therapy

PRODUCT	ACTIVE INGREDIENTS	ACTION
Eriderm (solution)	Erythromycin 2%	It suppresses the development of *C. acnes*, dries out and disinfects the skin. May cause local side effects such as skin irritation and redness, burning, dryness, flaking, itching.
Zerkalin (solution)	Clindamycin	It suppresses the development of *C. acnes*, dries and disinfects the skin. May cause local adverse reactions: skin irritation and redness, burning, dryness, flaking, itching. It is used to treat all forms of acne, either alone or in combination with other medicines.
Clindovit (cream)	Clindamycin	It inhibits the pathogenic microflora and stops the inflammation. It has to be used for a long time, i.e., for about three months. After a break, the therapeutic course may be repeated. It is often prescribed in combination with retinoids and/or benzoylperoxide.
Zineritis (lotion)	Erythromycin Zinc acetate	In addition to its bacteriostatic effect, it has a drying effect, suppressing sebum production. It is used in the treatment of mild to moderate acne. Sometimes the use of the drug causes increased skin dryness, and contact dermatitis develops.
Benzamycin (gel)	Erythromycin Benzoyl peroxide	It has an antibacterial effect, suppresses sebum production, promotes sebum cleansing, and prevents comedone formation. It is prescribed for mild to moderate acne.
Clensit C (gel)	Clindamycin Adapalene	It suppresses the development of *C. acnes*, and normalizes the epidermal cell division and keratinization processes, thus helping to reduce the number of inflammatory lesions, as well as open and closed comedones. Can cause redness, irritation, scaling.

Drugs of these groups are highly bioavailable, accumulating in the sebaceous glands, suppressing the development of pathogenic microflora in them. Systemic antibiotics are often prescribed as topical medications based on benzoyl peroxide and retinoids.

2.1.3. Glucocorticosteroids

Glucocorticosteroids (GCSs) are powerful anti-inflammatory agents, but their prolonged use impairs the epidermis's cellular renewal, the *stratum corneum* barrier's formation, and skin immunity. Moreover, taking systemic GCSs can provoke the development of acne (drug-induced acne). However, systemic GCSs at a dose of 2.5–5 mg in short courses may be indicated for severe inflammatory acne in women resistant to topical therapy.

2.2. Topical formulations

The cosmetic industry offers alternatives that are similar to medications in the mechanism of action and targets but are gentler and safer to use. If we are talking about long-term control of the process (which is precisely what we need in case of acne), then a gentle and effective strategy will be preferable. Especially in the initial non-inflammatory types, regular skincare helps prevent the development of acne and holds it until the regulatory mechanisms in the body are restored.

Generally, cosmetic products designed for oily skin (see Part IV, chapter 1) are also suitable for acne-prone skin. But there is also a specificity: several cosmetic formulations recommended for acne patients contain substances that are also used in medicines, for example, benzoyl peroxide, salicylic acid, and azelaic acid. Their concentration is usually higher in drugs, but the risks of adverse reactions are also higher.

2.2.1. Benzoyl peroxide

Peroxides are substances containing weakly bound atomic oxygen that is quickly released even at room temperature, causing the death of any microorganism. Everyone is familiar with the effects of hydrogen peroxide; when you apply it to the skin, bubbles form instantly — this is released atomic oxygen, which immediately combines into an oxygen molecule.

What is the value of peroxides? The fact that they have a detrimental effect on all festering bacteria is worthy of attention. Unlike antibiotics, peroxides never cause bacterial resistance. In addition, when they are applied to the skin, the oxygen-free environment of the comedone is quickly oxygenated, eliminating the opportunity for the growth of anaerobic bacteria such as *C. acnes*.

The range of peroxide-based products for treating acne patients is broad and includes dozens of trade names (**Fig. IV-2-2**). Formulations with benzoyl peroxide (Basiron AC, Effezel, Ugre-

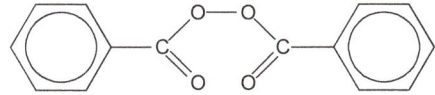

Figure IV-2-2. Benzoyl peroxide

sol) are over-the-counter drugs indicated for mild acne, the clinical picture of which includes comedones and a small number of inflammatory pimples. Benzoyl peroxide is also approved for use in cosmetic products (emulsions, gels, lotions, solutions). Its concentration in different products varies from 2 to 20%. But more does not mean better. Clinical experience has shown that the most effective preparations are those with a benzoyl peroxide concentration of 5–10%.

There is a downside: benzoyl peroxide causes skin irritation. To mitigate this side effect, benzoyl peroxide is included in a special base. Thus, acrylic copolymer formulations are thought to be better tolerated than traditional gels based on propylene glycol and carbomer. In addition, the acrylic copolymer can bind excess sebum, which is good since the skin is less "greasy" during the day.

All benzoyl peroxide-based preparations should be applied in a thin layer (ideally, they should be dotted on the lesion) only on the acne-prone skin that has been washed and thoroughly dried beforehand. Failure to observe this simple rule "diverts" the active oxygen to oxidize all kinds of impurities and skin grease, reducing the drug's effectiveness.

The product is applied once daily but regularly and without skipping for 2–3 weeks. More frequent use leads to severe skin irritation, which forces the patient to stop using the drug for a long time. We should start with the lowest concentration (5% gel) because even then, redness and scaling of the skin usually occur after a few days. These reactions are mild, and interrupting treatment if they occur is not recommended (after 7–18 days, the side effects disappear). After 7–10 days, it is possible to switch to a 10% preparation, which is recommended until the acne lesions have entirely disappeared. When using any benzoyl peroxide products, it should be remembered that they have oxidative power and discolor the hair when in contact with it.

It has been noticed that the effectiveness of benzoyl peroxide-based preparations increases dramatically if, before applying them, the skin is cooled for 1–2 minutes with an ice cube wrapped in a plastic bag (you can cover the bag with a thin cloth to avoid overcooling the skin). Perhaps this effect can be explained by the fact that benzoyl peroxide decomposes more slowly to molecular oxygen at lower temperatures, and therefore its action time is prolonged. In addition, ice almost immediately reduces tissue swelling which is inevitable in the inflammatory process, so the drug penetrates deeper into the sebaceous gland duct.

2.2.2. Salicylic acid

Salicylic acid is a phenol derivative (**Fig. IV-2-3**) and belongs to the keratolytic substances. The mechanism of keratolytic action is to break the intra- and intermolecular disulfide bonds that stabilize the 3D configuration of the protein (**Fig. IV-2-4**). As a result, the protein chain unfolds (denatures), and the protein ceases to perform its intended function.

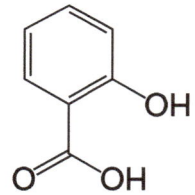

Figure IV-2-3. Salicylic acid

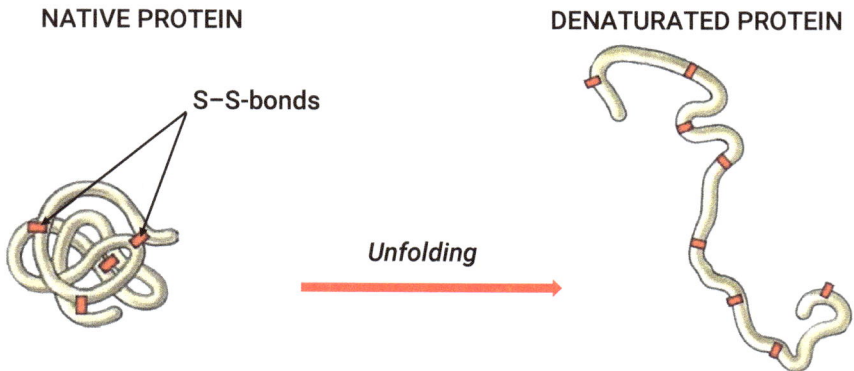

NATIVE PROTEIN

S−S-bonds

Unfolding

DENATURATED PROTEIN

Figure IV-2-4. The mechanism of action of the keratolytic is to break the stabilizing disulfide (–S–S–) bonds

Since disulfide cross-links are present in almost every protein, the keratolytic action will be non-specific, i.e., it reacts with any protein in its path. In the *stratum corneum*, these are keratin, proteins of cornified cell envelope, corneodesmosomes, enzymes of the *stratum corneum*, and shell proteins of microorganisms living on the skin.

If a keratolytic gets under the *stratum corneum*, its first targets are cell membrane proteins (receptors, pores). If the membrane is extensively damaged, the cell may even die, so keratolytics are characterized by cytotoxic effects. In this regard, **cosmetic keratolytics can only be used to work on the *stratum corneum* to exfoliate horny scales**.

In addition to the exfoliating effect associated with corneodesmosome denaturation, salicylic acid is characterized by two other beneficial effects in seborrhea and acne: bactericidal (due to the denaturation of microbial shell proteins) and sebostatic (due to the suppression of sebocyte maturation). Therefore, salicylic acid is prevalent in medicines and cosmetics (including peel formulations) intended for oily skin treatment and care. The concentration of salicylic acid:

- In non-washable topicals: up to 1%
- In salicylic masks: up to 2%
- In peel products: 15–30%

2.2.3. Azelaic acid

Azelaic acid (nonanedioic acid) is a dicarboxylic acid (**Fig. IV-2-5**). It is sometimes mistakenly linked to hydroxy acids, but it has nothing in common with them either in

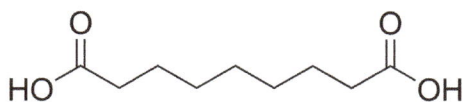

Figure IV-2-5. Azelaic acid

its chemical structure or properties or in its mechanism of action in the skin.

The action of azelaic acid on the skin consists of four primary effects — antibacterial, anti-inflammatory, comedolytic, and depigmenting — each having a specific mechanism of action. For example, azelaic acid can affect aerobic and anaerobic microorganisms' metabolism, enzymatic activity, and intracellular pH. This impact is associated with bacteriostatic action against many bacteria, including *C. acnes*. Interestingly, azelaic acid is highly tropic to *C. acnes*, and its concentration inside the bacterial cell can be 90 (!) times higher than in the environment.

The anti-inflammatory effect is partly due to a reduction in the number of *C. acnes* and partly due to direct inhibition of the release of pro-inflammatory mediators and ROS from the skin cells involved in the inflammatory response.

Its comedolytic effect manifests because azelaic acid affects sebum lipid production in sebocytes and reduces the production of long-chain fatty acids that contribute to acne. In addition, azelaic acid inhibits the proliferation of basal keratinocytes by inhibiting DNA synthesis and decreasing their maturation rate, reducing the respiratory function of mitochondria. As a result, when using drugs containing azelaic acid, the *stratum corneum* becomes thinner, and signs of hyperkeratosis are less pronounced. This is a good prevention of closed comedones.

DNA inhibition under the influence of azelaic acid is also recorded in melanocytes, which explains the depigmenting effect. In the context of post-inflammatory pigmentation prevention, typical for post-acne, the anti-inflammatory effect of azelaic acid is also essential.

All of these effects are beneficial in acne treatment, which is why azelaic acid is used at different stages of the disease. Clinical improvement occurs after an average of 2–4 weeks of treatment. In rare cases (in the first 1–2 weeks of therapy), skin irritation and burning sensation may occur.

The therapeutic concentration of azelaic acid is 15–20%. It is part of such well-known drugs as AcneStop, Acne-Derm, Azelex, Azogel, Azix-Derm, Finevin, Finacea, Skinoren, and Skinoklir.

Azelaic acid is often found in skincare products for patients with acne, rosacea, and melasma. Its concentration can be as low as 10%, but it is often combined with other beneficial active ingredients like antioxidants, salicylic acid, and niacinamide.

2.2.4. Non-comedogenic emollients

Make-up can worsen acne if it contains ingredients stimulating the comedone formation. These substances do not clog the ducts, as previously thought, but trigger complex biochemical processes that lead to blockage of the duct by horny scales and inflammation.

Of course, acne patients are tempted to buy cosmetics with the promising claim that they are non-comedogenic. Unfortunately, this claim does not give a full guarantee of safety. The thing is that not all the ingredients that can be found in cosmetics are tested. But even if we assume that all cosmetic ingredients have undergone additional testing for comedogenicity, we must keep in mind that:

1. The results obtained on rabbit ears (on which the comedogenic effects of cosmetics are usually studied) are not always reproducible on human skin.
2. Comedogenic action of ingredients depends on their degree of purification, concentration, and presence of other substances.
3. Individual skin sensitivity to comedogenic ingredients is highly variable: what is non-comedogenic for one person may cause clogging of pores in another.

Comedogenic substances are primarily emollients that soften the skin. Comedogenic compounds include isopropyl palmitate, isopropyl myristate, butyl stearate, isopropyl isostearate, decyl oleate, isostearyl neopentanoate, isostearyl stearate, myristyl myristate, and cocoa butter.

But petroleum jelly and paraffin, disproving popular opinion, do not provoke comedones. Cetyl alcohol, stearyl alcohol, and sodium lauryl sulfate (surfactant often found in cleansers) do not clog pores on rabbit ears either. But this does not mean that sodium lauryl sulfate can be used without hesitation for oily skin and skin with compromised barrier properties because its irritating effect on the skin is associated with damage to its barrier structures.

2.3. Cosmetic products and aesthetic procedures

In addition to special cosmetics for daily hygiene and care of acne-affected skin, there are other aesthetic methods (**Table IV-2-3**) that, if integrated into acne management program, accelerate the healing, reduce the risk of post-acne complications, and improve the psycho-emotional state. Let's focus on the most popular ones.

Table IV-2-3. Skincare treatments for acne prevention and treatment

OBJECTIVE	TOOLS AND TREATMENTS
Removal of comedones (deep cleansing)	• Comedone extraction
Removal of surface impurities (superficial cleansing)	• Cosmetic cleansers • Brossage • Desincrustation • Ultrasonic cleaning • Gas–liquid peeling
Normalization of the keratinization process	• Chemical peeling
Restoration of the local regulation of sebum production	• Cosmetic products (phytoestrogens, retinol and its esters, azelaic acid, zinc preparations) • Mesotherapy (regulatory peptides) • Placentotherapy • Platelet-rich plasma (PRP) therapy
Modulation of skin immunity, anti-inflammatory effect	• Cosmetic products (regulatory peptides, nicotinamide, beta-glucan, pro- and prebiotics, topical carboxytherapy) • LLLT (low-level laser therapy using radiation in the red and infrared parts of the spectrum) • Mesotherapy (regulatory peptides, amino acids, nucleic acids, antioxidants, and anti-inflammatory substances)
Antibacterial effect	• Cosmetic products (herbal extracts with antiseptic action — chamomile, calendula, gammamelis, arnica, etc.), essential oil of tea tree, benzoyl peroxide • Ozone therapy • Phototherapy (blue light)

2.3.1. Cleansing

Oily skin needs regular deep and superficial cleansing. By cleansing the skin of comedones, excess sebum, and impurities, we create more favorable conditions for therapeutic work.

Deep cleansing (comedone extraction)

Deep cleansing means removing (extracting) comedones. No matter what we do, no matter what drugs or cosmetics we use, if the sebaceous glands are clogged, the inflammation issue is a matter of time. Therefore, regular clearing of the sebaceous gland ducts is essential.

Extraction begins with the formation of a passage through which the gland's content can escape. The classic method of removing closed comedones (**manual extraction**) is to open the cavity of a clogged pore with a thin needle. Then the skin near the orifice is gently pressed with the fingers. An instrument with one or more holes called an Unna spoon (**Fig. IV-2-6**) can be used for extrusion. In the case of large cysts, it may be necessary to curettage the cavity to

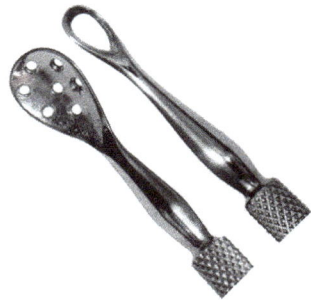

Figure IV-2-6. Unna spoon extractors

remove the pus. After cleansing, the skin is treated with antiseptics for several days to avoid infection around the removed comedone.

As for **vacuum extraction**, it understandably cannot guarantee the complete extraction of comedones, and the risk of damaging the surrounding tissue remains high. In addition, it cannot be used in couperosis and increased vascular fragility.

Removal of comedones provides rapid clinical improvement. This simple method gives the most splendid result both in the initial stages and in the later treatment phases. Of course, for nodules and cysts, you still have to resort to surgical methods to evacuate the pus.

Superficial cleansing (exfoliation)

The surface of oily skin is more contaminated than that of skin with normal or reduced sebum production. It's not just excess sebum and dirt buildup but also conglomerates of horny flakes that contribute to this effect.

Special cleansers with mild surfactants and pH 4.0–5.0, used both in the procedure and at home (see Part IV, section 1.2.1), have been developed to clean oily and acne-prone skin. They can be in milk, foam, or mask form. For exfoliation, you can use enzymatic cleansers — solutions or liquid gels containing enzymes that break down organic substances (proteins, fats, carbohydrates).

For superficial cleansing of the skin with acne, the following treatments are also used:

- **Brossage:** mechanical exfoliation with special brush heads. It is indicated in the initial non-inflammatory stages of acne.
- **Desincrustation:** pre-wetted with an alkaline solution, skin is treated with a galvanic current. This involves a chemical reaction of saponification of fatty acids, which loosens greasy conglomerates and facilitates their subsequent removal with water.
- **Ultrasonic peeling:** loosens the *stratum corneum* and exfoliates horny scales through the mechanical action of ultrasonic waves. The method is perfectly integrated into any cosmetic protocol, conducted after make-up removal, cleansing milk, and combined with toning. The general effects of the ultrasonic wave (anti-inflammatory, antibacterial, defibrotic, reparative and regenerative, hydrating) during the session are poorly expressed because the ultrasonic waves do not penetrate the depth of tissue and are reflected from the skin surface.
- **Gas–liquid peeling:** peeling is achieved with compressed gas and an aqueous solution of various active substances. During the treatment, the skin is treated with finely dispersed droplets, which hit the skin surface at high speed and "knock out" the upper horny scales, helping them leave the skin.

Proper daily cleansing at home is essential for oily and acne-prone skin. But periodically, it is necessary to carry out a deeper cleansing, which should be done in a skincare specialist's office. The main goal is to avoid traumatizing the *stratum corneum*, as the skin barrier is already very weakened.

2.3.2. Chemical peeling

Acne-prone skin is susceptible to damage and infection because its defenses are compromised at the *stratum corneum* level and the local immune system. Being a damaging procedure, chemical peeling can worsen the already poor skin's ability to defend itself and resist external influences. Inflamed skin must be treated with particular care. In this case, the chronic inflammatory fire will reignite and cause even more damage, including the appearance of pigmentation spots (post-acne pigmentation).

In addition, inflammatory mediators, particularly histamine, increase sebum production. This makes the need for anti-inflammatory measures in acne therapy and the contraindication of damaging procedures even more apparent.

As for the non-inflammatory acne (comedonal), chemical peeling is acceptable, but only if it is superficial and non-traumatic.

More information about chemical peel products and treatments can be found in the *Chemical Peeling in Cosmetic Dermatology & Skincare Practice* book.

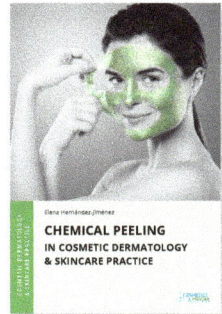

Elena Hernández Jiménez

CHEMICAL PEELING
IN COSMETIC DERMATOLOGY
& SKINCARE PRACTICE

Keratolytic peeling
The following keratolytic substances are used:
1. Salicylic acid and liposalicylic acid
2. Resorcinol
3. Trichloroacetic acid (TCA)
4. Phenol

Today, the use of TCA and phenol is prohibited because of their high cytotoxicity and ability to penetrate the *stratum corneum* rapidly. **Salicylic acid**, on the other hand, although a derivative of phenol, passes poorly through the *stratum corneum*; its main action is concentrated on the surface and within the *stratum corneum* (see Part IV, section 2.2.2). The concentration of salicylic acid in the peel formulation is between 15% and 30%. Salicylic peeling is recommended for seborrhea, seborrheic dermatitis, as well as non-inflammatory and mild inflammatory forms of acne.

Resorcinol is another phenol derivative. It is also a keratolytic agent, but it has a higher chemical activity and penetration capacity than salicylic acid. Resorcinol is much less commonly used than salicylic acid because of its higher irritant potential. It can be found in disinfectants at a concentration of around 1%, which is not enough for peeling, but is sufficient to disinfect the surface. Resorcinol is included in Jessner peels at a concentration of about 14%. In addition to resorcinol, salicylic acid (14%) and lactic acid (14%) are present in the classic Jessner peel formulation. The active ingredients are dissolved in ethanol (95%). In modified Jessner peels, resorcinol is replaced by citric acid or glycolic acid, for example, to reduce the risk of side effects. Jessner peels are mainly used to treat post-acne skin damage.

The current trend is to combine salicylic acid with alpha hydroxy acids (AHAs) in one formulation thus significantly expanding the therapeutic possibilities of salicylic acid.

The exfoliation of horny masses occurs during the keratolytic peeling session: a whitish plaque (frost) appears on the skin — it is formed by denatured proteins and detached horny scales. Sometimes there can be a light scaling for a few days after the treatment, which is a consequence of the inactivation of the horny layer enzymes by the keratolytic agent. However, this secondary scaling is not always present; it depends on the concentration of the keratolytic agent, duration of the chemical peel exposure, skin condition, and post-peel care.

Acid peeling

Peel treatment performed by acutely acidifying the skin is called an acid peeling. The active components of acid peel products (acid peels) are AHAs. These substances contain two functional groups — hydroxy (–OH) and carboxy (–COOH) (**Fig. IV-2-7**) — and most of them are water-soluble.

Acid peels are aqueous solutions or gels. The aim of acid peel is the shock violation of the pH gradient through the *stratum corneum*, resulting in an abrupt halt of all enzymes responsible for keratinization and desquamation (**Fig. IV-2-8**). The exfoliating power of an acid peel is related to its pH: the lower it is, the stronger the skin scaling. To stop the effect of an acid peel, the pH must be restored, and a neutralizer is used for this purpose.

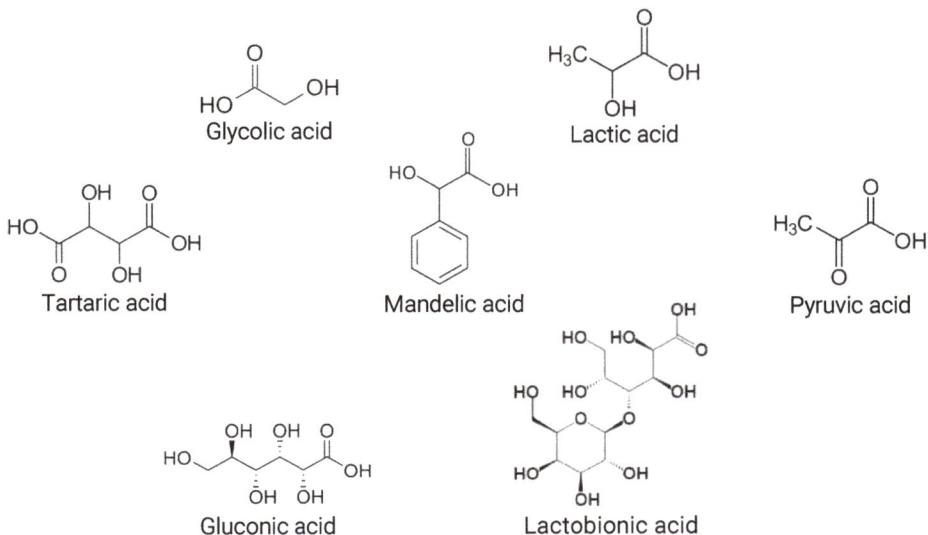

Figure IV-2-7. Alpha and polyhydroxy acids in cosmetic products for oily and acne-prone skin

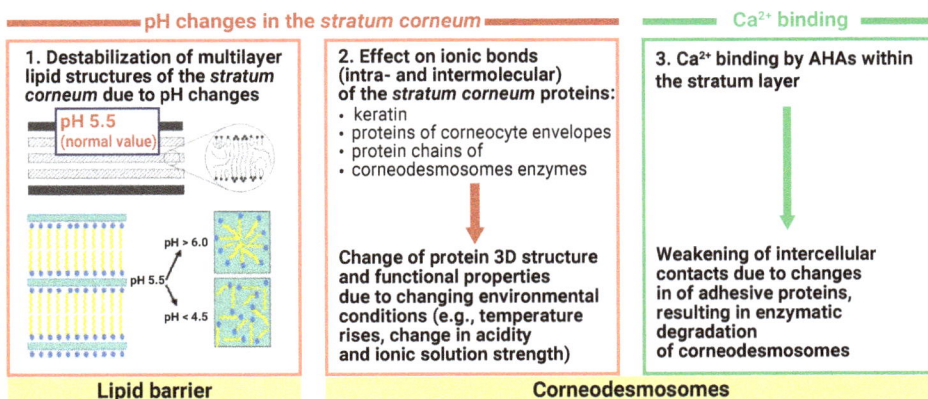

Figure IV-2-8. Mechanism of action of AHAs

The result of enzymatic failure in the *stratum corneum* is the formation of abnormal corneocytes and intercellular lipid structures. The skin tries to shed them as quickly as possible to make space for new normal barrier structures. This does not happen immediately; visible desquamation is noticeable a few days after the treatment.

AHAs are frequently used in acne treatment due to their moisturizing ability (e.g., lactic acid saturates the *stratum corneum* with water). This property is required in case of oily skin, which is also dry. The diagnosis of "oily dry skin" at first glance sounds strange. But it is true: skin that "suffocates" from too much sebum often suffers from a lack of water in the *stratum corneum*. In acne, the water-holding and barrier structures of the *stratum corneum* are severely compromised and, as a result, the *stratum corneum* is poorly hydrated. Lactic acid, a component of natural moisturizing factor (NMF), penetrates the *stratum corneum* and retains within it the water molecules necessary to maintain the structural and functional integrity of the skin barrier.

The following AHAs are the most popular in clinical practice:

- **Polyhydroxy acids** — lactobionic and gluconic acids, as well as gluconolactone, a derivative of gluconic acid — "work" similarly. These large molecules do not penetrate beyond the *stratum corneum* but concentrate in it and moisturize it owing to the binding of water molecules.
- **Almond acid**, known for its bactericidal and keratolytic properties, is found in formulations for oily and acne-prone skin.
- In formulations for post-acne skin, **tartaric acid** is often used as it lightens the skin and increases its elasticity.
- **Glycolic acid**, as the smallest among hydroxy acids, easily penetrates through the *stratum corneum* (if it is damaged, as in acne, penetration occurs very quickly). It reaches the living skin layers, which react with inflammation. Therefore, glycolic peels are not indicated for acne. It is acceptable to use low-concentration (<10%) glycolic acid formulations with a pH of at least 4–4.5 as home care to soften the *stratum corneum* and keratinized sebaceous gland orifices. Still, such products often contain glycolic acid in combination with other AHAs (usually lactic and salicylic acids).
- An alternative to glycolic peels for mild acne characterized by open and closed comedones can be pyruvic acid peels, called Red Peels, because of the intense red color. **Pyruvic acid,** a highly lipophilic keto acid that quickly penetrates the sebaceous glands, is characterized by its keratolytic, sebostatic, bacteriostatic, restructuring, and depigmenting action. In the skin, pyruvic acid can be converted to lactic acid. Comedonal and papulopustular

forms of acne can be treated with 50% pyruvic acid (the pH is about 1–2). According to the literature, undesirable reactions and complications following pyruvic acid peeling are rare. Epidermal detachment (epidermolysis) can occur if the patient uses topical retinoids or undergoes mechanical peeling (dermabrasion, scrubs) right before the chemoexfoliation procedure. The risk of postinflammatory hyperpigmentation, perioral dermatitis, and urticaria after pyruvic acid peeling is low. Such reactions occur more often in patients that cannot refrain from scratching the skin in the peel-treated area. Despite the promising clinical efficacy, most pyruvic acid-containing products have limited efficacy in treating acne (especially its inflammatory forms) because they have a pronounced irritating effect due to the low pH. A special base that provides more even penetration of pyruvic acid into the skin and reduces the mobility of protons in the peel solution helps make the peel less irritating.

Enzymatic peeling

Hyperkeratosis observed in seborrhea and acne is associated with a decrease in the proteolytic activity of the *stratum corneum*. Desquamation of horny scales is provided by proteolytic enzymes (proteases) working in the middle and superficial layers of the *stratum corneum*. If desquamation is insufficient, corneocytes cannot leave the skin in time, and the *stratum corneum* thickens. In such cases, external help by applying a solution with enzymes similar to the proteases of the *stratum corneum* is appropriate and effective.

Enzymatic peels usually include proteases of plant origin: **papain** (derived from papaya juice), **ficin** (from fig leaves and fresh fig shoots), and **bromelain** (from pineapple juice). Some products on the market contain an enzyme of microbial origin **subtilisin** or modified enzymes, such as **cross-papain**.

Enzymatic peels are typically in aqueous solution form, but can also be gels. The question of enzyme stabilization is critical. That is why heating during the production process is prohibited and care must be taken when choosing other substances to add to ready-to-use formulations: alcohol, emulsifiers, and keratolytic agents inactivate the enzyme. It is necessary to maintain the pH of the finished preparation at the level of 5.5–6.0. Preserving the structure of the enzyme is essential, as is its protection from microorganisms because it is a protein molecule that is a convenient substrate for most microbes. Therefore, all enzyme formulations must contain preservatives.

A few words about the peculiarities of the enzymatic peel. Before the first treatment, it is necessary to perform an allergy test because the enzyme is a protein, and proteins, as we know, are the most allergenic of all organic compounds.

As the enzymes need water to work, the peel must be applied to cleaned and hydrated skin. While the preparation remains on the skin, covering it with a warm damp towel is recommended. This is done so that the water from the product does not evaporate, and the skin remains sufficiently moisturized. Exposure time varies from 10 to 30 minutes for different preparations and skin conditions (it is essential to follow the manufacturer's recommendations). Afterwards, the skin should be thoroughly washed with warm water to remove the product. Neutralization is not required even if the enzymatic peel contains AHAs because the pH of the product is above 4. Finally, a moisturizer is applied to the skin, which may include components of NMF. When going outside after the treatment, sunscreen should also be applied at this stage.

Enzymatic peeling is a gentle treatment, after which there are no adverse reactions in the form of persistent redness or swelling. On the contrary, the skin after the treatment is smoother, acquires a beautiful shine, and looks refreshed. Therefore, the enzymatic peel is commonly known as an express procedure "for going out." But it can also be carried out as a series of 5–8 treatments. For oily skin, seborrhea and non-inflammatory forms of acne, enzymatic peeling can be performed 2–3 times a week. In case of extensive inflammation, this treatment is not recommended since the proteolytic activity of the *stratum corneum* is increased in the inflamed area. Using an external enzymatic preparation can provoke an aggravation.

Retinol peeling

Acne is treated with topical and systemic retinoids (see Part IV, section 2.1.1). Retinol peels (with the retinol concentration not exceeding 10%) are not indicated because they can provoke an exacerbation of the underlying disease.

2.3.3. Phototherapy

Phototechnologies have been used for therapy since the beginning of the 1990s. The accumulated experience shows that using light as monotherapy only leads to partial and temporary remission. Ideal candidates for phototherapy are patients for whom topical therapy improves the condition only by 40–50% and who do not want to take oral systemic medications. Combining phototherapy and topical drugs makes it possible to achieve complete remission in these patients.

The phototherapy targets are:

1. **Cutibacteria.** *C. acnes* synthesize porphyrins. After absorbing blue light (in the 407–420 nm wavelength range), these molecules are excited, followed by the release of ROS, which leads to irreversible membrane damage and death of the bacterial cell. However, blue light cannot penetrate the skin deeply enough to kill all the bacteria settled in the sebaceous glands.
2. **Sebocytes.** Blue light (415 nm) has been shown to inhibit the proliferation of sebocytes and red light (630 nm) to inhibit sebum production in a sebocyte cell culture. Combined blue and red light exposure is therefore recommended for acne therapy (Jung Y.R. et al., 2015).
3. **Immunocytes.** Low-intensity red and infrared (IR) light penetrates deeper than blue light and can reduce inflammation by modulating cytokine release from macrophages (Li W.H. et al., 2018).
4. **Water.** High-energy near-IR radiation heats water to a depth of 400–500 µm, warming the dermis and having bactericidal, anti-inflammatory, immunomodulatory, and sebostatic effects.
5. **Hemoglobin in erythema areas.** In the papulopustular acne with a predominance of superficial inflammatory lesions, "vascular" lasers emitting in the yellow–green range are used. This exposure promotes the completion of the inflammatory process.

Both low-intensity and high-energy lasers are used for acne and post-acne treatment. As for the use of weak light-emitting diode (LED) sources, which are positioned on the market for so-called chromotherapy (color treatment) and emit light in the blue and red spectral ranges, their effectiveness has not been proven.

Low-level laser (light) therapy (LLLT)

LLLT in the red and infrared parts of the spectrum is often used, as it is characterized by good penetrating ability and sufficiently physiological effect on the skin. LLLT with power from 0.1 to 100 mW/cm² does not cause visible skin destruction. Its therapeutic results are associated with photochemical effects on biological structures. LLLT increases phagocytic activity of macrophages, positively influences the functions of lymphocytes and neutrophils, stimulates reparative and trophic processes, activates microcirculation, normalizes the proteolytic activity of enzymes, increases blood oxygen transport function, and stabilizes cell membranes. The following variants of LLLT are used:

- Local laser therapy (irradiation directly to the lesion)
- Peripheral irradiation of the lesion with a focused beam
- Laser acupuncture
- Reflex exposure to the projection area of regulatory organs
- Intravenous laser irradiation of blood
- Autotransfusion or transcutaneous laser irradiation of the blood
- Photophoresis

High-energy laser therapy

Application of pulsed dye lasers (PDLs) with low energy and a wavelength of 625–740 nm leads to a significant improvement in skin condition (a 53% reduction in the number of lesions vs. 9% in control) after 12 weeks. Laser radiation in this range can have a direct bactericidal effect and can modulate the immune response to infection. Besides, it affects the formation of comedones and follicle maturation, improving the keratinization process. A PDL has been successfully used to treat congestive erythema and dyschromia, which complicate the course of the papulopustular type of acne vulgaris.

Currently, electromagnetic radiation in the IR range is approaching the forefront of acne therapy. Particular attention is paid to radiation in the visible part of the spectrum — violet, blue, green, yellow, orange, and red wavelengths.

Radiation in the violet (380–420 nm) and blue (420–485 nm) range generated by the argon laser penetrates deeper (90–150 μm) than ultraviolet (UV) light and gives a moderate bactericidal effect. Despite the pronounced antibacterial activity of violet and blue light, the impact of radiation is realized in the upper part of pilosebaceous follicles. The greatest follicle infestation with *C. acnes* is observed mainly in comedonal and superficial papulopustular acne. Therefore, these easily progressing acne forms are the main indication for the application of IPL or laser radiation in the violet and blue range without additional photosensitizers.

Radiation in the green (500–565 nm, KTP laser), yellow (565–590 nm, copper vapor laser), and red (625–740 nm, dye laser) ranges penetrates deep enough (280, 450, and 550 µm, respectively) and can have a damaging effect on *C. acnes* in the hair follicle funnel. In patients with papulopustular acne, as the depth of inflamed follicles usually exceeds 2 mm, it is more effective to use red light with a wavelength of 630–1064 nm. Nevertheless, bactericidal properties of radiation in these ranges are noticeably weaker than in the violet and blue ones. To enhance the bactericidal effect, they are combined with radiation in the violet range. Topical or oral photosensitizer precursors (such as 5-aminolevulinic acid, 5-ALA) selectively absorbed by *C. acnes* and keratinocytes and metabolized into protoporphyrin IX are also used. Irradiation of protoporphyrin IX results in ROS production, aiding in the destruction of target cells and bacteria. This method is called **photodynamic therapy (PDT)** (see Part IV, section 2.3.4).

When irradiated with IR laser (1500–3000 nm), the follicle funnel is heated, and most *C. acnes*, as we have already written, are located deeper. So, IR radiation has neither bacteriostatic nor direct bactericidal action. Its main target is water, which is present in the sebaceous gland due to inflammation and perifollicular edema (usually, there is almost no water in sebaceous glands). When exposed to high-intensity IR light, the water heats up, damaging the gland. The positive effect of such radiation on acne is evident, as the sebaceous gland production activity is reduced.

On the other hand, its effect can negatively affect the normal skin function by raising the temperature above 50 °C and provoking side effects, including pain. To minimize the adverse effects, it is preferable to use infrared lasers with a temporary sebum-suppressive impact on the sebaceous glands. The devices are designed so that the wavelength, as well as the pulse duration and intensity can be regulated, thus controlling the strength of the effect. In addition, many lasers are equipped with cooling technologies. They protect the epidermis from excessive heating without influencing the photothermal effect in the deeper layers of the skin. For example, a 1450-nm laser with a cryospray, leaving the epidermis intact, heats tissue to a depth of about 200–500 microns, where most sebaceous glands are located.

According to clinical practice, the neodymium-doped yttrium aluminum garnet laser (Nd:YAG) emitting in the invisible near-IR spectral range (1064 nm) is the most preferable in acne therapy. This radiation is minimally absorbed by the upper skin layers and reaches the deeper skin layers. Acne treatment with Nd:YAG laser is based on the phenomenon of homogeneous photothermolysis at a depth of up to 4 mm. The method is pathogenetic due to direct sterilization of inflammation foci, i.e., the bactericidal effect is produced not only on *C. acnes* but practically on any microorganism. There is a normalization of microcirculation due to coagulation of vessels in the inflamed area and stimulation of trophic processes due to enhanced revascularization. In addition, the sebaceous glands are also affected, which leads to their damage and, consequently, to the reduction of production activity. The method is applicable for any form and degree of acne.

Applying light technologies in acne management allows for steady positive dynamics during the disease. Microcirculation is improved, inflammation and bacterial growth are significantly reduced, and post-acne manifestations are also lessened. The efficiency of acne phototherapy largely depends on the spectrum influencing the critical targets.

In mild acne, these targets are primarily *C. acnes*, abundantly present in the sebaceous gland ducts and containing endogenous photosensitizers (porphyrins).

In severe acne, the planning of acne phototherapy can take one of two directions: (1) application of an exogenous photosensitizer before exposure to radiation in the visible spectral range, or (2) use of near-IR radiation (Nd:YAG laser, 1064 nm), which sterilizes the focus, eliminates inflammation, and significantly reduces sebum production by photothermic effects across the entire thickness of the dermis.

2.3.4. Photodynamic therapy (PDT)

In photodynamic therapy (PDT), the targets are photosensitizers applied to the skin. Photosensitizers traditionally used in dermatology are aminolevulinic acid (ALA) and its lipophilic derivative methyl aminolevulinic acid (MLA). When applied topically, these compounds penetrate keratinocytes and are converted to protoporphyrin IX, accumulating in the epidermis and pilosebaceous complexes. Subsequent skin irradiation leads to photoactivation of protoporphyrin IX and cell damage. In addition, ALA and MLA induce porphyrin production directly in *C. acnes*, increasing their sensitivity to blue light. Unfortunately, after the treatment, erythema, swelling, pain, burning sensation, scaling, and even hyperpigmentation (especially in patients with darker skin) occur. These unpleasant side effects limit the use of PDT in clinical practice.

With the advent of a new generation of chlorine-based photosensitizers derived from microalgae, the problem of adverse reactions was solved. Today this method is increasingly used in inflammatory acne therapy and post-acne treatment, delighting skincare specialists and their clients (patients) with excellent clinical results (Gelfond M.L. et al., 2017). The photosensitizer gel is applied to the skin and then irradiated with 662-nm light (**Fig. IV-2-9**).

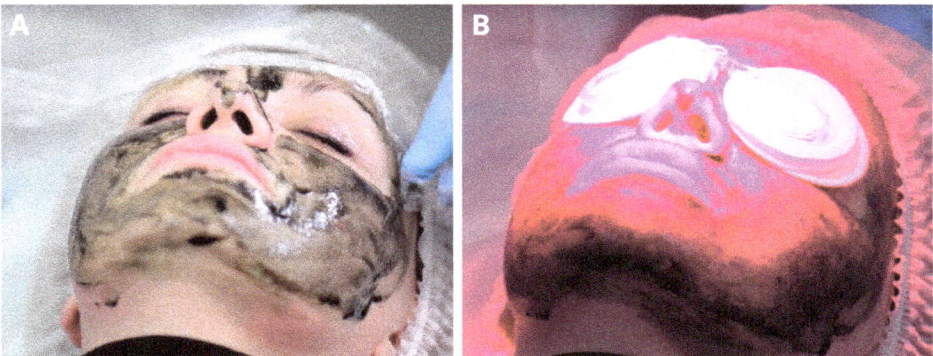

Figure IV-2-9. Photodynamic therapy: A — photosensitizer application and exposure for absorption; B — light irradiation

In PDT, photosensitizers are used to enhance the effectiveness of phototherapy: in dermatology — aminolevulinic acid (ALA) and methyl aminolevulinic acid (MLA), in aesthetics — chlorophyll derivatives.

2.3.5. Plasma shower

The method is based on treating the skin's surface with low-temperature plasma. This is ionized air with reactive forms of oxygen and nitrogen. They cause irreversible damage to the cell walls of all microorganisms, which explains their disinfecting effect and usefulness in acne therapy.

Several variants of plasma devices that are available on the market differ in the way the plasma is obtained and delivered to the skin. The technology called "plasma shower" (**Fig. IV-2-10**) is the most suitable for oily skin and acne. The name reflects the way the plasma is delivered — in the form of low-energy thin "jets" resembling a shower. They do not injure the skin but cause intense oxidative stress in its surface structures — the hydrolipid mantle and the *stratum corneum*. As a result, all microorganisms within the treatment zone die. Though it will not be directly damaged, the *stratum corneum*'s permeability will change due to the oxidative processes in the intercellular lipid structures. If water-soluble active substances are applied to the skin immediately after the treatment, their penetration through the *stratum corneum* will improve. This strategy can be used to introduce anti-inflammatory molecules or immunomodulator peptides indicated for oily skin.

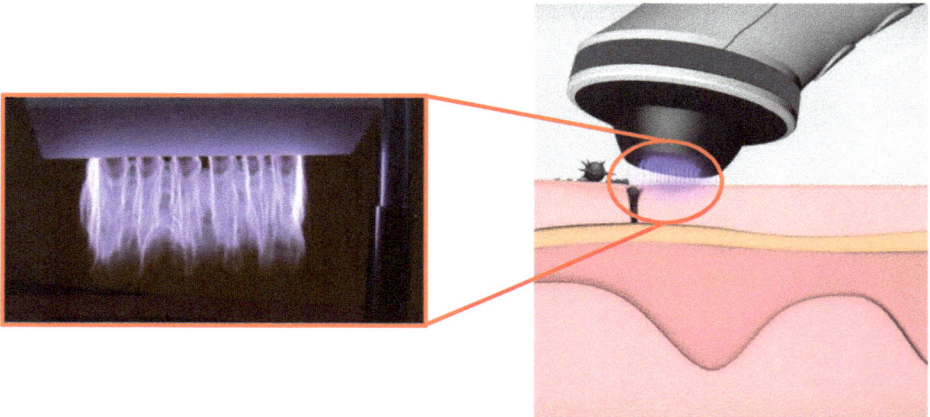

Figure IV-2-10. Plasma shower

2.3.6. Intradermal injections

Injecting active substances directly into the skin (intradermally) by a needle allows the necessary substances to be delivered with high precision and in the right quantity. However, the skin is traumatized by the subsequent launch of reparative processes accompanied by inflammation. In the case of acne, the trauma can provoke an aggravation and eruption of new inflammatory lesions.

Mesotherapy

Until recently, even non-inflammatory acne was considered a contraindication for mesotherapy. Today, there are injectable solutions with anti-inflammatory properties on the market, designed for acne patients' skin. They belong to a new generation of mesotherapy products that contain modulators of immune reactions and the optimal set of substances necessary for cellular metabolism. Such substances include, for example, the nucleic acid complex. In addition to the fact that nucleotides are the building material for synthesizing the cell's DNA and RNA, they have been found to have signaling functions. They directly affect the synthesis of pro- and anti-inflammatory cytokines via cell receptors and stimulate angiogenesis. Some synthetic regulatory peptides, antioxidants (thioctic acid, glutathione), trace elements (selenium) can help to cure the initial inflammation and single pimples. In post-inflammatory pigmentation on seborrheic skin, mesopreparaions with salts of glycyrrhizic acid from licorice root are suitable.

Sometimes, such special mesopreparations can be used even in papulo-pustular acne. The products are introduced by the gentlest technique into the epidermis to minimize trauma to the skin.

Placenta injections

Curacen and Melsmon, two Japanese products approved for intradermal administration, are obtained from the human placenta by multistage purification. Their formulas include a composition of low-molecular-weight regulatory peptides, amino acids, polyunsaturated fatty acids, and macro- and microelements. They are injected into the subcutaneous fatty tissue to create a depot from which the substance is gradually released. It is not necessary to create a depot directly in the inflamed skin; it can be done on the unaffected areas, thus avoiding skin traumatization. The clinical effect at the local level is to stop the inflammation and lighten the pigmentation quickly.

This method yields good clinical results in treating late acne in women, even at the stages with inflammatory lesions, as well as in the complex treatment of post-acne.

Ozone therapy

The bactericidal properties of ozone O_3 (an allotropic modification of oxygen, consisting of three oxygen atoms, an unstable oxidizing agent) are known, and its injection directly into the acne lesions has long been practiced. In general, ozone therapy has an effect, but we must keep in mind the complexity — effects on other targets of pathogenesis must necessarily complement antimicrobial action. In this regard, we should pay attention to organofluorine compounds.

Organofluorine compounds

Organofluorine compounds (OPCs) are organic compounds with all hydrogen atoms replaced by fluorine atoms.

There is a fascinating history associ ated with OPCs. They were first mentioned in the 1980s as potential blood substitutes. One of the OPCs representatives — perfluorodecalin, an active ingredient of the Perftoran solution (**Fig. IV-2-11**) — was considered a blood plasma substitute. Like hemoglobin, it is capable of binding and releasing oxygen. However, hemoglobin is inside red blood cells, which cannot always penetrate microcapillaries, especially in trauma. In this respect, OPCs are advantageous because they are much smaller than red blood cells and can reach the most remote areas, which is especially valuable in ischemia.

OPCs are used in emergency medicine, cardiology, and transplantology. They have recently begun to be used in dermatology and aesthetic medicine. When injecting perfluorodecalin into

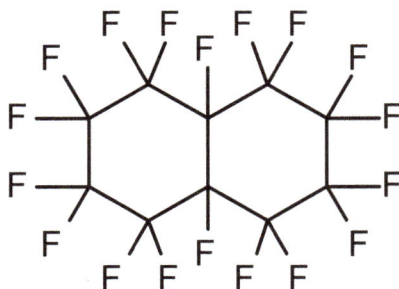

Figure IV-2-11. Perfluorodecalin

the soft tissues, there is a good and fast effect of improving microcirculation. As a result, edema and congestion disappear, and skin regeneration improves. Any skin damage, whether physical trauma or pathology, is an indication for the use of OPC injections. Acne is one of them, including the active inflammatory stage.

OPCs can capture inflammation mediators and flush them out of the damaged area, which is especially important in the case of chronic inflammatory processes. OPCs also have bactericidal properties associated with fluoride being a strong oxidant.

As a result, injectable OPC preparations can be considered an alternative to antibiotics with additional important favorable properties in the form of improved microcirculation and regenerative potential. These properties allow OPCs to relieve acute and chronic inflammation associated with inflammatory acne (Korneeva R.V., 2018, 2019).

2.4. Nutraceuticals

We have already talked about how to balance nutrition (including nutraceuticals) to avoid triggering acne (see Part IV, section 1.1.2). **All of these recommendations are also appropriate for acne.**

Probiotics, magnesium sulfate, pyridoxine, zinc gluconate, omega-3 polyunsaturated fatty acid complex, antioxidants — the benefits of using these substances in nutraceuticals for oily skin and skin with acne are proven, and the mechanisms of action are generally straightforward. To this list, we add two more compounds that have only recently begun to be included in nutraceuticals for skin with active acne.

Diindolylmethane (DIM) is a natural substance in certain vegetables such as broccoli, cauliflower, and white cabbage. DIM was previously better known as a natural substance that influences signaling pathways and can regulate cancer cell division, apoptosis, and angiogenesis. DIM is used in drugs to treat hyperplastic and cancerous conditions, such as prostate cancer, early-stage breast cancer, cervical dysplasia, proliferative thyroid disease, gastrointestinal diseases, and hormonal imbalances. Not so long ago, it was discovered that DIM could be used to treat active acne due to its ability to bind to (but not activate) androgen receptors like estrogen does. Thus, DIM has an anti-androgenic effect, reduces sebum production, and prevents excessive proliferation of sebocytes and keratinocytes.

There are already products with DIM on the market specifically for acne skin. DIM can be combined with retinol and/or antioxidants in these formulations.

Another substance worth considering in acne prevention and treatment is **nicotinamide adenine dinucleotide hydride (NADH)**. It is a natural compound participating in the respiratory metabolism of the cell. Its action involves various biochemical pathways, one of which is the transport of electrons along the respiratory chain in the mitochondria and the synthesis of adenosine triphosphate (ATP). ATP is the universal fuel for cells and is consumed in various biochemical reactions involving the synthesis and decomposition of substances. Cell viability and activity are directly related to how efficiently the cell replenishes its energy reserves. In chronic diseases, including inflammatory conditions (such as acne), there is often mitochondrial insufficiency, in which ATP production is reduced. This is where oral NADH supplementation is especially indicated.

On the one hand, cells in the injury and inflammation area exhibit oxygen deficiency and poor gas exchange due to impaired microcirculation. On the other hand, their mitochondrial enzymes deteriorate, and the cells' ability to synthesize ATP decreases. Therefore, it is worth thinking about improving mitochondrial function and restoring microcirculation. In this respect, NADH turned out to be just right. Today there are both topical and oral formulations based on a stabilized form of NADH on the market, and their clinical effects — antioxidant, immunoprotective, cytoprotective — have been scientifically proven. However, in acne therapy, the oral form is more effective because it has a systemic effect and makes a noticeable contribution to the normalization of regulatory mechanisms at the level of the body as a whole. The skin will feel it and will respond with gratitude (Birkmeyer G.J., Lazuk A.V., 2018).

2.5. Causes of acne treatment failure and the importance of psychological correction

Despite a wide choice of topical medicines and skincare products for acne-prone skin, a dermatologist often hears the following phrase from a patient seeking help: "I have tried everything — creams, lotions... Nothing helps. Maybe I need a pill?"

The lack of effect from topical treatment indicates the need for systemic therapy, which is characterized by a more pronounced effect on the pathological process and the whole body, such as the teratogenic effect of systemic retinoids, digestive disorders caused by antibiotics, etc. Therefore, it is essential to understand the reasons for the "ineffectiveness" of a particular formulation for topical therapy in each clinical case before abandoning it and moving on to systemic treatment. (We do not consider cases where systemic therapy is initially indicated for the patient.)

2.5.1. What does "ineffective treatment" mean?

According to evidence-based medicine, ineffective treatment boils down to the ineffectiveness of a particular medication. Ineffective medications are those the therapeutic efficacy of which has not been proven by reliable clinical trials conducted in full compliance with evidence-based medicine (Greenhalch T., 2009).

However, the ineffectiveness of treatment (including topical therapy) is a broader concept than the ineffectiveness of a single drug. The physician sometimes doesn't get the desired result even from medications with proven efficacy. Why? At least four reasons can be identified:
1. Unproven therapeutic efficacy of the prescribed topical formulation
2. Unreasonable prescribing of a topical formulation
3. Violation of the rules of use by the patient
4. Lack of trust between the doctor and the patient

Let us discuss each aspect in more detail.

2.5.2. Unproven therapeutic effectiveness of the prescribed topical formulation

Therapeutic efficacy is the ability of a drug to produce the desired results, which is confirmed or refuted by clinical studies. The design of the study itself is essential — where and by whom it was conducted, sample size, methodology, availability of direct evidence of clinical benefit, etc.

When collecting and analyzing the information about a drug, the physician will benefit from the knowledge of evidence-based medicine, skills in searching for scientific data, and the ability to critically evaluate information provided by the representatives of pharmaceutical companies (Nikolaeva N.N., 2019). It is no secret that some companies promote their products using results from clinical trials which do not meet evidence-based medicine requirements. When communicating with commercial representatives, ask them about (Greenhalch T., 2009):

- Safety (S) — the likelihood of severe side effects (including distant ones) caused by the drug
- Tolerability (T) — can be evaluated by comparing the frequency of discontinuation of a given product with its most popular competitor
- Efficacy (E) — the most critical aspect of this criterion is to compare the drug to the one you currently prefer
- Price (P) — should include direct and indirect costs

The combination of these criteria is referred to as STEP. Always be guided by these criteria when analyzing information about a medicine!

As for cosmetic products and aesthetic treatments, the evidence base is even more limited, but there are still conscientious manufacturers who conduct efficacy and safety studies, even if they are not as large-scale and lengthy as studies conducted on medicines. They are mostly pilot studies with a small sample of volunteers or retrospective studies that analyze the clinical experience already gained. Still, they can generally serve as a guide for selection.

2.5.3. Unreasonable prescribing of a topical drug

When deciding on the treatment method for a particular patient, the physician should be guided by the accepted clinical guidelines and current standards of medical care pertaining to the relevant patient profile. At the same time, we should not forget the primary tool physicians have at their disposal — clinical thinking, which provides an adequate diagnosis, and the best ways of treatment, rehabilitation, and prevention. Unfortunately, as Trisha Greenhalgh writes in her book *The Basics of Evidence-Based Medicine*, "very few recommendations are based on evidence-based medicine" (Greenhalch T., 2009).

The main requirements for reasoning in any domain, and thus medicine, are a high level of abstraction and knowledge of the laws of logic. For example, one of the laws of formal logic, the law of sufficient reason, requires that every statement be justified. Evidence-based medicine is designed to help the physician make the right decision using scientifically proven findings. Please don't take for granted the loud assurances of salespeople and sales representatives; understand the mechanism of action of the product/treatment offered and find the logical connection between it and the promised result!

2.5.4. Violation of the rules for the topical medication application by the patient

The patient plays a vital role in achieving treatment results. After all, the patient must comply with the doctor's recommendations regarding the frequency of application of external medication, the duration of external therapy, etc.

Accordingly, we recently surveyed 54 acne patients to gain insight into their attitudes toward topical therapy. For this purpose, we designed the questionnaire *Attitude of an Acne Patient Toward Topical Medications*. The analysis of the questionnaire results showed that 78% of the respondents consider using a single (without systemic drugs) topical therapy ineffective. To the question "Did you discontinue the use of the topical drug prescribed by your doctor?" 81% of participants responded positively. In 57% of cases, the reason for failing to comply

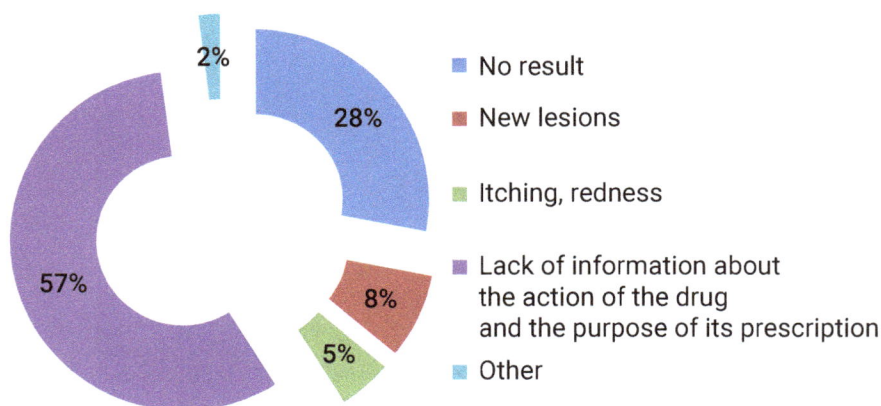

Figure IV-2-12. Reasons why patients discontinue the use of acne medications prescribed by a doctor

with the doctor's advice was a lack of information about how the medication works and why the patient needed it (**Fig. IV-2-12**).

In addition, in most cases, those surveyed did not adhere to the rules of application and storage of a the prescribed drug: only 26% of participants adhered to the number of applications during the day, 17% to the duration of application, 20% to the sequence of application, and 30% to the rules of its storage at home.

These survey results show patients' inadequate (often negligent) attitude to topical acne therapy (81% of the survey participants refused the treatment prescribed by the dermatologist!). Of course, a more objective picture of the patient's attitude towards the treatment can be obtained using special tests. Nonetheless, even the findings based on a relatively small patient sample regarding topical acne treatment should worry doctors. After all, doctors play a key role in shaping patients' attitudes towards treatment and their disease.

Here, another problem arises: the lack of trust and cooperation between the doctor and the patient. In this case, the doctor–patient relationship acquires a predominantly formal character.

2.5.5 The formal nature of the doctor–patient relationship

Unfortunately, modern medicine treats the patient as an object to be influenced rather than a subject that should be engaged in the treatment plan and its execution. Although a doctor informs the patient about the state of health and planned treatment, the patient seems to decide independently by signing many documents. Still, in most cases, patients do not feel responsible for their health condition, are not fully aware of their role in the treatment process, and tend to shift the responsibility for their health and the treatment outcomes to the doctors.

Yet, such formal communication mode is necessary to comply with the legal norms of medical care. However, the interpersonal aspect of communication between doctor and patient is no less critical for the treatment process. Thus, the doctor should rely not on worldly psychology in contact with the patient but on clinical psychology.

It is necessary to understand that patients tend to have a subjective picture of the illness which is autoplastic and has its structure (**Fig. IV-2-13**).

In addition, patients have different attitudes toward their disease. In pertinent literature, several types of patient attitudes toward

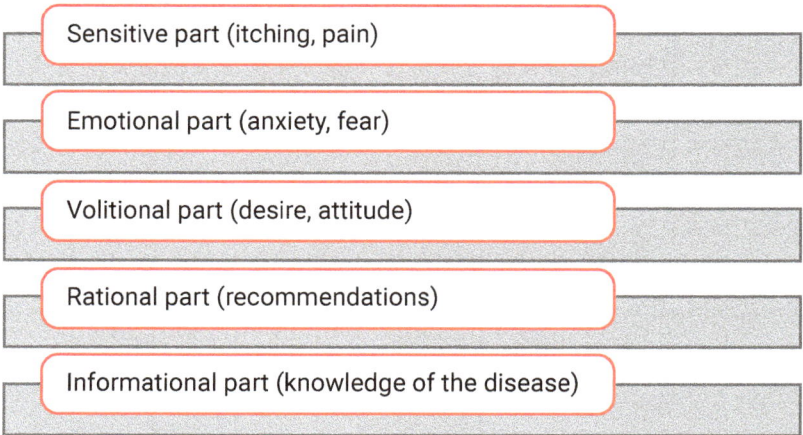

Sensitive part (itching, pain)

Emotional part (anxiety, fear)

Volitional part (desire, attitude)

Rational part (recommendations)

Informational part (knowledge of the disease)

Figure IV-2-13. Autoplastic disease pattern

the condition have been identified, including: nosophilic, nosophobic, hypochondriacal, dismissive, etc.

It becomes clear that, for example, the treatment will be the same if the patients treat their disease neglectfully. Therefore, when dealing with such a patient, a doctor needs to emphasize the seriousness of the illness and its possible consequences (for a clinical case and a discussion of a doctor's approach to care, see section 2.6.3).

For a doctor, it is equally important to be aware of how the patient experiences his or her illness (**Fig. IV-2-14**). For example, the patient in a stage of active adaptation (typically lasting 3–5 days) asks the doctor a wide range of questions about the illness and treatment. Thus, if the doctor calmly answers all these questions during this period, the patient adapts more successfully and contributes to the treatment process.

This is especially true for patients with acne. It has long been known about the psychosomatic nature of acne and the reactive depression that occurs in such patients, as well as about the personality features of acne patients (high anxiety, inadequate self-esteem, aggressiveness, suicide risk, etc.). It is no coincidence that acne in patients with

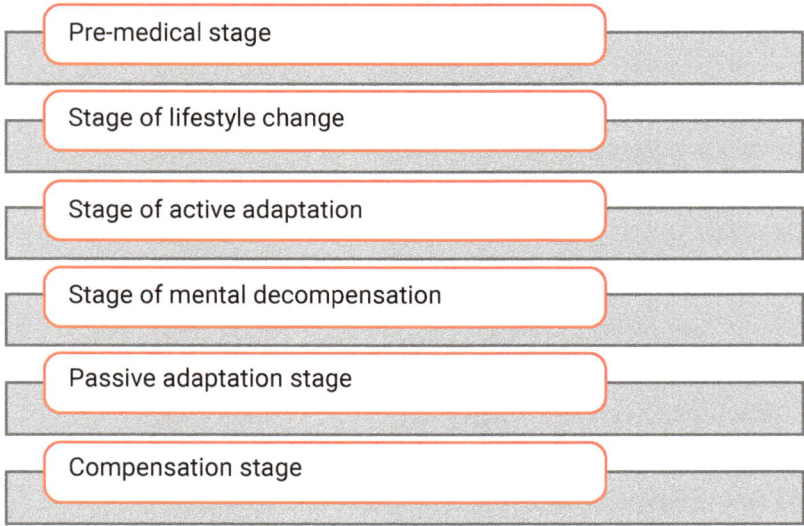

Pre-medical stage

Stage of lifestyle change

Stage of active adaptation

Stage of mental decompensation

Passive adaptation stage

Compensation stage

Figure IV-2-14. Stages of patient's experience of the disease over time

pronounced psycho-emotional disorders and negative attitudes toward the disease is an indication for systemic treatment.

In this regard, the physician's task is not to inform the patient about the disease and the required external medication but to build a constructive relationship with the patient based on trust and cooperation. This is the most critical factor influencing the success of treatment of this long-lasting disease.

2.6. Combined approaches in the treatment of moderate to severe acne (clinical examples)

In treating a polyethiological disease such as acne, the best results can be achieved only through different methods — medications, physiotherapy, aesthetic, nutraceutical, and psychotherapeutic. In the early stages, acne can be controlled by cosmetic and device-based treatment modalities; in later stages, inclusion of drug and physical therapy becomes necessary. In each case, treatment needs to be individualized, as demonstrated in the following examples featuring a few clinical studies and case studies.

2.6.1. Lasers and retinoids

A combination of low-dose isotretinoin and laser treatment may be a potentially effective option. However, there are concerns that this drug increases skin sensitivity to light and stimulates cell proliferation, which could theoretically provoke hypertrophic or keloid scars after injury. Typically, patients taking isotretinoin are advised not to undergo surgery or dermatologic procedures. However, several studies indicate the safety of dermabrasion (on a small area of skin) in patients taking oral isotretinoin (Bagatin E. et al., 2010).

For laser treatment, it should be noted that non-ablative fractional lasers use IR radiation for deep penetration into the skin, selectively heating the dermis and not affecting the epidermis. They are considered a safe and effective skin improvement method requiring minimal recovery time. In many prospective studies, non-ablative lasers have been used to treat mild to moderate acne and post-acne scars (Darne S. et al., 2011). It is believed that the light "trauma" of the skin after such treatment is much less pronounced than after IPL.

Second, spontaneous keloid formation after isotretinoin rarely occurs in practice (Dogan G., 2006). One review lists nine studies of combined treatment with oral isotretinoin and laser, including four cohort studies, three case series, and two clinical cases. Only two studies mention keloid scars after combination therapy: in one case, the patient received isotretinoin at a dose of 60 mg/day, and in the other, an unknown amount of the drug was administered (Zachariae H., 1988).

Recently, a team of experts from the United States analyzed articles published between 1982 and 2017 to assess the likelihood of complications after light therapy in patients receiving isotretinoin. No substantial evidence was found to support the need to delay laser procedures for patients taking this medication (Spring L.K. et al., 2017). The American Society for Dermatologic Surgery (ASDS) published a consensus recommendation for physical and surgical interventions during and after taking isotretinoin. The findings do not support the need to delay chemical peeling or non-ablative laser treatments in patients currently or previously taking isotretinoin (Waldman A. et al., 2017).

Clinical experience is essential in overcoming concerns and developing specific protocols. Here are a few examples.

Low-dose isotretinoin and fractionated Er:glass laser (1550 nm) in the treatment of moderate to severe acne

An interesting study was conducted by Chinese researchers (Xia J. et al., 2018). It is known that for Asian patients, the comfort dose of retinoids is lower than for European patients. Based on the authors' clinical experience, many Asian individuals with acne cannot tolerate the 20 mg/day doses of isotretinoin because of adverse severe mucosal reactions, including cheilitis and dry eye syndrome, as well as skin dryness and flaking. Reducing the oral dose of isotretinoin minimizes the severity of side effects, but at the same time, the therapeutic effect is diminished.

Therefore, the authors tested whether combination therapy using low-dose isotretinoin (10 mg/day) and a 1550 nm non-ablative fractionated laser could produce a synergistic effect and reduce the likelihood and/or severity of adverse reactions. To do this, they conducted a prospective monocenter randomized controlled trial in which half of each participant's face was treated with the laser (side A), and the other half was not treated and served as a control (side B). The sides were randomly assigned. Twenty-four people over 18 years of age with phototype II–IV and moderate to severe acne were selected for the work. Each patient received a low dose of isotretinoin for 30 to 45 days before laser treatment (baseline acne scores were 6 to 12, with an average of 10.6).

In a single pass, treatment was performed using a 1550 nm fractionated Er:glass laser. Each patient underwent three treatments at 1-month intervals and exposure at the level of the middle dermis. The laser was operated in low-energy mode (20 mJ/cm², 100–169 points per area) to reduce the risk of hypertrophic and keloid scars. Side A was cooled with ice packs for 30 min. Patients received antibiotics and a collagen face mask for 1–2 weeks after the sessions to restore the skin — moisturizing cream and avoiding sunlight after laser treatment was also recommended.

Eighteen people (mean age 24.16 years; range 18–38 years) with a mean acne duration of 4.7 years (range 2–8 years) completed treatment. They were also followed up for nine months after therapy. After three sessions, significant improvement was recorded on both sides of the face. The mean acne severity score decreased from 10.6 to 5.8 on the control side of the face and from 10.4 to 3.5 on the treated side, and this difference was statistically significant. The number of comedones decreased significantly on side A compared to side B. The number of papules and nodules did not differ significantly between the sides. There was a marked improvement in superficial and deep rectangular post-acne scars, but chipped and rounded scars were unaffected.

The most common complications were dry mouth and cheilitis, which all patients tolerated well. Only one participant complained of excessive dryness of the eyes, which had to be treated with special drops. Reddening of the face was noted in 55.5% of the patients. Serum levels of liver enzymes, cholesterol, and triglycerides were normal. The laser-treated side of the face had no signs of hypertrophic scars and keloids. Uncomfortable sensations during treatment included pain

(100% of patients), heat (100%), erythema (94.5%), and edema (88.9%), which subsided spontaneously within 24 h. The remaining effects disappeared within 1–3 days. No patients reported any long-term complications, and all were satisfied with the results of complex therapy.

Interestingly, after completion of therapy, five patients requested erbium laser sessions on both sides of the face. Long-term follow-up of all participants is ongoing to evaluate the long-term effects of this comprehensive treatment.

Laser therapy against systemic isotretinoin in the treatment of conglobate acne

A 16-year-old patient sought treatment from a dermatologist in February 2018 for multiple painful lesions on the face, back, and shoulders (**Fig. IV-2-15**). Previous treatment which lasted two years, including inpatient treatment with systemic antibacterial therapy, topical antiseptics, retinol acetate, and physical therapy, was ineffective. The result was a temporary slight decrease in inflammation with

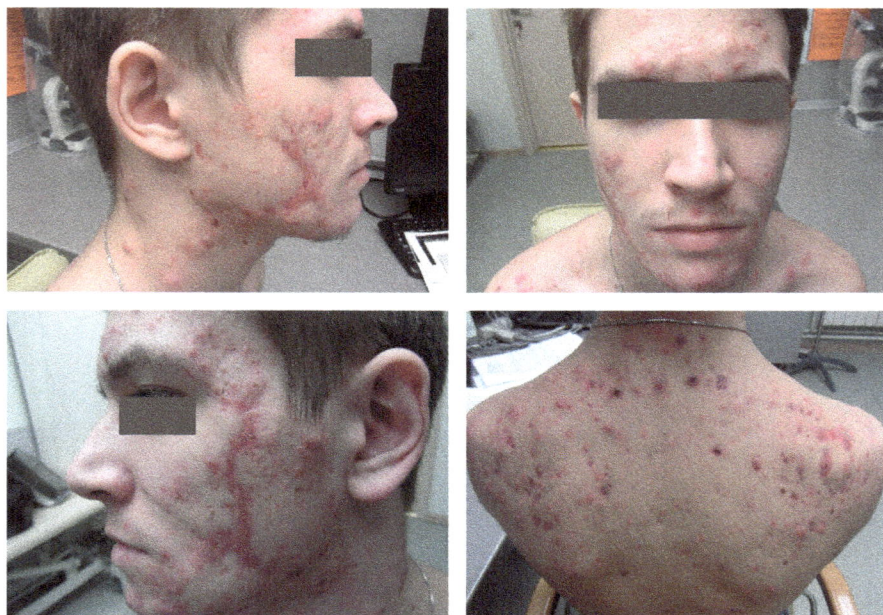

Figure IV-2-15. Patient before treatment (photo: Kalashnikova N.G., Albanova V.I.)

further aggravation and spreading. Concomitant diseases: chronic gastritis, out of exacerbation.

The pathological process was widespread and inflammatory, with localization in the face, neck, back, chest, and upper half of the shoulders. The skin of the face was oily, with multiple open and closed comedones, small follicular papules, and large confluent nodules with a yellowish discharge of thick pus. Large, dense, red, tightening, and deforming irregular-shaped scars with superficial tissue tension, and pearlescent sheen occupied a large surface area of the cheeks. It spread to the sub-chin area of the neck. A small number of atrophic scars up to 1 cm in diameter with a relief depression up to 0.5 cm was also observed. Multiple large nodules and infiltrates, some with areas of melting in the center and secretion of creamy pus and formation of thick bloody crusts, were located all over the back and external surface of the shoulders. Many retracted circular scars were observed at the sites of resolved eruptions up to 4 cm in diameter, along with purplish-blue spots and single comedones.

Diagnosis: severe conglobate widespread acne in the acute stage.

Therapy: oral isotretinoin (0.5 mg/kg/day), external clindamycin gel twice a day, sensitive skincare (washing gel, facial moisturizer, shower gel, and body lotion), diet, blood chemistry monitoring after two weeks of treatment, and then every three months.

The persistent course of the pathological process served as an indication for increasing the dose of systemic isotretinoin after three months to 1 mg/kg/day, after which persistent positive dynamics with a decrease in the number of newly appearing inflammatory lesions and disappearance of old lesions were noted. By October 2018, the isotretinoin dose was reduced to 0.25 mg/kg/day with persistent results and rare isolated infiltrates in the face and back (**Fig. IV-2-16**).

Considering the pronounced facial scarring changes, which significantly worsened the patient's psycho-emotional state, the physician decided to perform a cosmetic treatment of the existing changes against the background of continued oral administration of isotretinoin. The patient was referred for a consultation with a cosmetic surgeon to decide on the possible use of laser treatments.

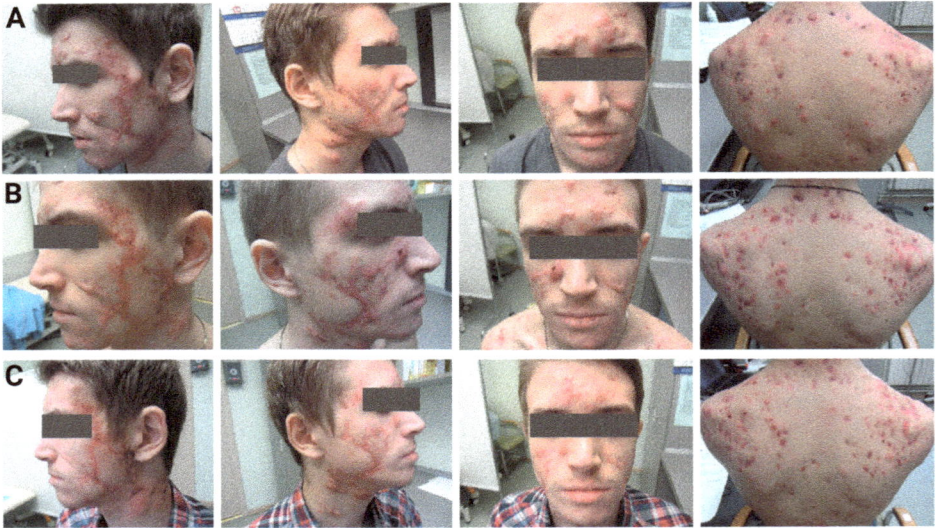

Figure IV-2-16. Patient in the treatment dynamics with systemic isotretinoin: A — after 2 weeks of therapy; B — after 2 months; C — after 8 months (photo: Kalashnikova N.G., Albanova V.I.).

The rationale for the early initiation of laser treatment in this particular patient included:

- Data from the outlined reviews overwhelmingly show that the risks of hypertrophic scarring, keloid formation, delayed wound healing, and pigmentation are not significant when laser treatments are performed against a background of systemic isotretinoin
- Presence of an aesthetic defect of a pronounced degree in the open area, which is an indication for the use of laser treatment
- Psycho-emotional aspect, which plays an essential role in adolescence in all spheres of life
- The current stable course of the inflammatory process with rare occurrences of single infiltrates

Considering the large lesion area, the scars with a tendency to hypertrophic growth (rising above the surrounding skin, dense, bright red scars with a shiny surface, and occasional itching sensation), the continued use of systemic isotretinoin (16 mg/day) and the associated risk of adverse events, we formulated the following principles to improve treatment safety:

- Aesthetic laser treatment was offered as a part of the study with prior familiarization of the patient and his parents with the probable risk of complications and the signing of appropriate informed consent
- Mandatory constant dynamic observation of the patient with examinations at two-week intervals to monitor and detect signs of complications on time
- Starting treatment with a small test area followed by tissue response assessment and, in case of positive dynamics, gradual expansion of the treatment area
- Use of silicone-based topical agents in the area of laser treatment, which is included in the current recommendations for the prevention of pathological scarring
- Constant use of sunscreens for exposed areas and restriction of active insolation during the whole course of treatment

The therapy was carried out in stages.

Stage 1

Treatment was initiated in the face using the Nd:YAG/KTP vascular laser to coagulate vessels in areas with a tendency to hypertrophic growth and the presence of subjective sensations in the form of intermittent itching (**Fig. IV-2-17**).

Induced hypoperfusion under theinfluence of yellow–green laser radiation leads to a decrease in the cellular activity of fibroblasts (Nast A. et al., 2012; Koike S. et al., 2014), causes intracellular changes (reduction of TGF-β1 expression), which suppresses fibroblast proliferation and collagen synthesis, and stimulates cytokine release with activation of collagen lysis and induction of fibroblast apoptosis (Nast A. et al., 2012; Poetschke J., Gerd G., 2016). Clinical efficacy in treating immature scars with vascular lasers is manifested by relief of subjective sensations, reduction of redness expression, reduction of density and volume of excess tissue, improvement of relief, and elimination of surface tension.

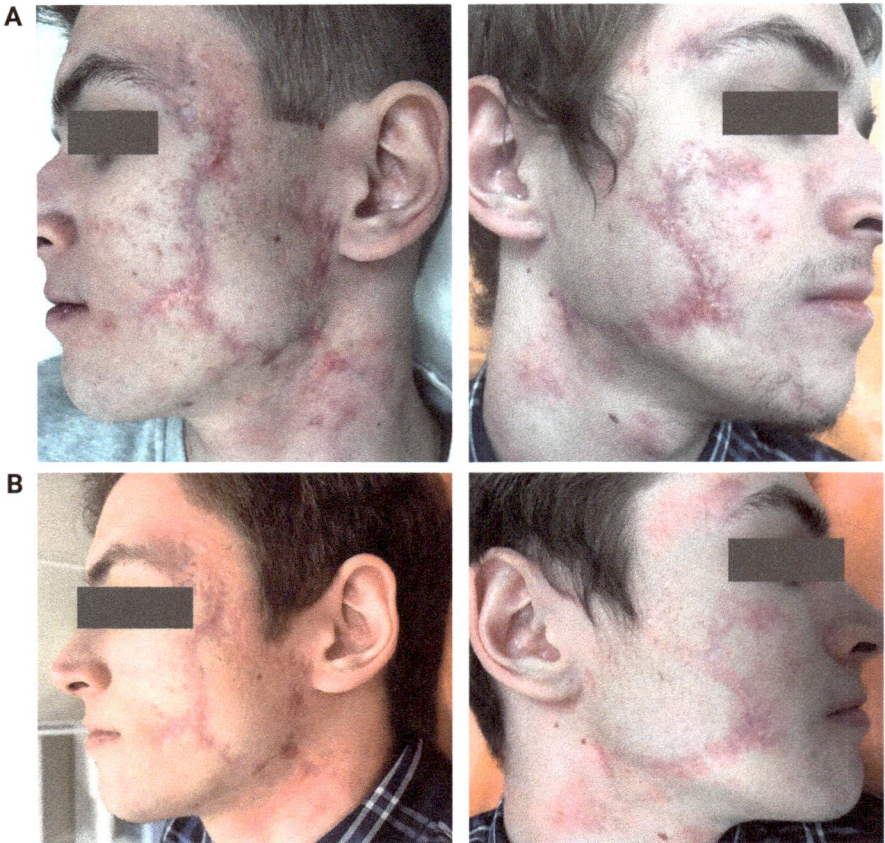

Figure IV-2-17. Patient before and after laser coagulation of the vascular component in facial scars: A — before the laser therapy; B — after 4 sessions of laser coagulation with Nd:YAP/KTP (photo: Kalashnikova N.G., Albanova V.I.)

In this patient, the preferential choice of the vascular laser was based not only on the need to achieve external positive dynamics but also on the importance of reducing the risk of scarring against the background of taking systemic isotretinoin. A small 2×2 cm area in the parotid region on one side was treated during the first session. After evaluation of the therapy efficacy after two weeks, which was manifested as the reduced itching intensity and lower density of treated tissues, the procedure was carried out with the treatment of all the scars tending to hypertrophy in the face and neck area.

Laser radiation parameters:
- Nd:YAG/KTP laser (1079/540 nm)
- Diameter of the light spot: 3 mm
- Pulse frequency: 2 Hz
- Energy density: 14–28 J/cm^2

A total of four sessions were performed with an interval of 2–3 weeks. The subjective sensations disappeared, the severity of hyperemia decreased from bright red to pink, and the elevated areas were depressed to the level of the surrounding skin. They became less dense.

Stage 2

The next stage of laser treatment aimed to remodel the scar tissue and optimize the skin relief. The method of choice was spatially modulated ablation using an Er:YAG laser (2940 nm) with the SMA module — a micro-ablative technology with interferential micro traction (Alcolea J.M. et al., 2014; Volkova N.V. et al., 2017). The peculiarity of this method is the small size of ablation zones (50 µm) with depth at the level of the *stratum corneum*. They serve as the source of acoustic waves which propagate into deep layers and realize the main therapeutic effect due to their interference with a local increase in power, leading to mechanical micro-traumatization of tissue structures. Depending on the energy parameters, spatially modulated ablation has a stimulating effect: at 1–3 J/cm^2, it activates neocollagenogenesis; above 3 J/cm^2, it destroys excess collagen. The clinical therapeutic effect of its use in scar revision manifests in optimizing surface relief, tissue density, and color by smoothing the transition boundaries between healthy skin and scar tissue.

In December 2018, we performed the 1st session with the use of spatially modulated ablation on a test area (2×2 cm in the parotid region on one side) on the face with monitoring of the recovery period, which did not differ from its usual course; delayed healing was not noted. In two weeks, positive dynamic changes were recorded, after which treatment was performed on the whole face and scars in the neck area.

Laser radiation parameters:

- Er:YAG laser (2940 nm)
- SMA module: 5 mm
- Pulse frequency: 2–3 Hz
- Energy density in areas with a tendency to hypertrophy: 3.7 J/cm² on atrophic scars —2.4 J/cm²

After three sessions of spatially modulated ablation on scars in the face and neck area with a pronounced therapeutic effect (**Fig. IV-2-18**) without adverse reactions, the treatment area expanded to the upper back and its entire region with post-inflammatory defects.

By November 2019, seven sessions of spatially modulated ablation were performed in the facial area, four sessions on the upper back, and two sessions on the lower back at one-month intervals. The patient continues oral administration of isotretinoin at a dose of 8 mg/day and is monitored by a dermatologist. No adverse reactions were noted during 11 months of laser treatment.

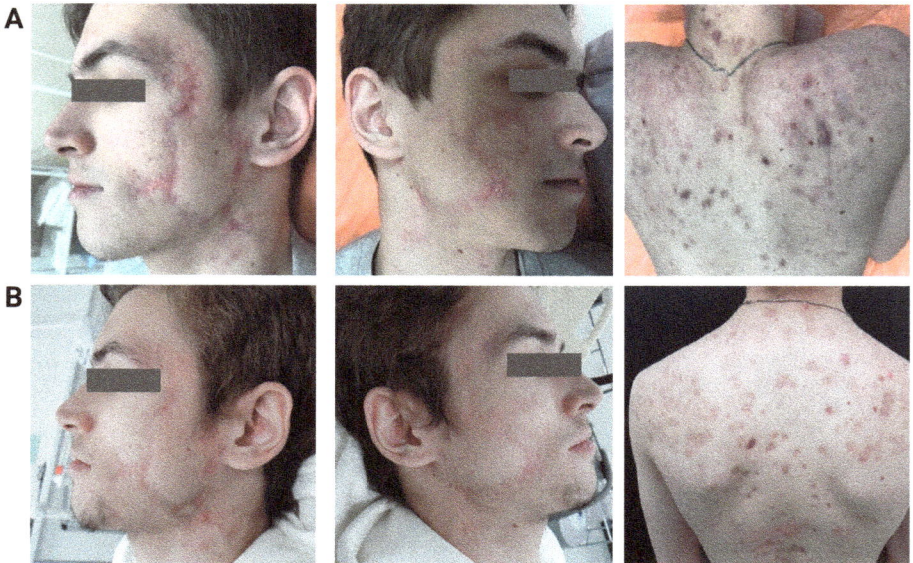

Figure IV-2-18. Patient before and after the course of Er:YAG/SMA laser treatment: A — before; B — after 7 sessions on the face and 4 sessions on the back (photo: Kalashnikova N.G., Albanova V.I.)

The patient tolerates the treatment well and expresses high satisfaction with the obtained results, not only from the aesthetic point of view but also, to a great extent, in terms of improved self-esteem, better mood, adaptation to the social environment, with reduction of withdrawal and more active communication with his peers.

Thus, during 1.5 years of treating a patient with a severe degree of disseminated conglobate acne characterized by a persistent course, we managed to achieve a stable remission of inflammation, an expressed aesthetic result due to the post-acne treatment, and a positive impact on the psychological status, which is especially important in the adolescent period.

The continuity of therapy made it possible to implement a combined treatment approach using laser therapy against the background of oral isotretinoin administration. This therapeutic combination induced no adverse reactions and helped to optimize the treatment time and obtain positive results (**Fig. IV-2-19**). Moreover, early laser treatment of post-acne scars not only did not result in pathological scarring but also allowed us to control areas with a tendency for hypertrophic growth with subsequent formation of normotrophic scars. Oral administration of isotretinoin in combination with space-modulated ablation allowed us to avoid the probable aggravation of the inflam-

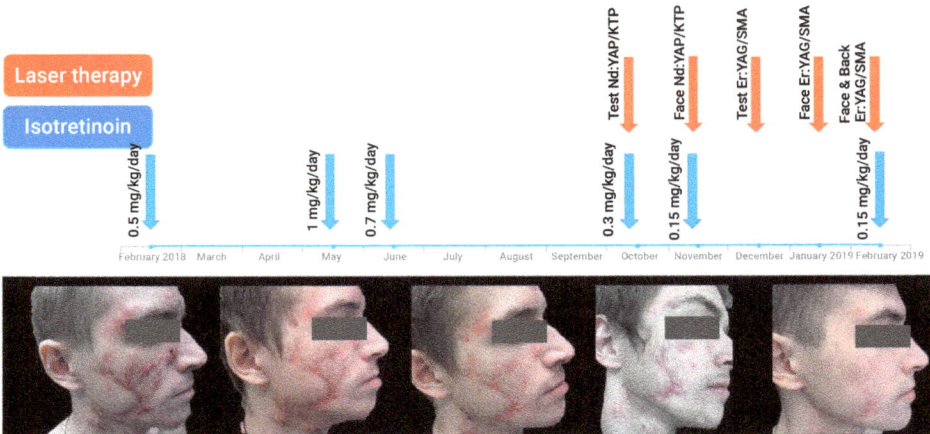

Figure IV-2-19. Dynamics of the clinical picture of a patient with conglobate acne during combined therapy with systemic isotretinoin and laser treatment (photo: Kalashnikova N.G., Albanova V.I.)

matory process after isotretinoin withdrawal. The patient is scheduled to continue treatment under the supervision of a dermatologist and aesthetician.

2.6.2. Laser therapy in acne resistant to medication

An exciting study concerning laser therapy for acne was conducted by American dermatologists (Bakus A.D. et al., 2018). The 1064 nm Nd:YAG laser emits infrared light that penetrates deep into the dermis and reaches the pilosebaceous complex, almost without affecting the epidermis. It is known that such lasers can also be effective in treating post-acne scars, but devices with different pulse durations give slightly different results. The authors decided to study the clinical efficacy, safety, and long-term effects of the combination of long-pulse and QS Nd:YAG (1064 nm) lasers in drug-resistant forms of acne. They performed a retrospective study involving 20 patients (15 women and 5 men) with moderate to severe acne. Participants ranged in age from 17 to 47 years (mean age 26 years), Fitzpatrick skin phototypes I–VI). Many of the volunteers responded poorly or not at all to topical and oral retinoid regimens. Pregnant women and patients who had taken photosensitizing drugs, systemic antibiotics and retinoids in the past six months did not participate in the study.

Therapy. Photographs of the affected areas were taken before the therapy was initiated. Patients were advised to stop local treatment two weeks before the first session and throughout the course of laser treatment.

The handle of the 1064-nm long-pulse Nd:YAG laser (Lyra, Cutera, USA) was equipped with a skin-cooling sapphire tip, which the doctor used to guide the ultrasound gel applied to the skin. This protected the epidermis from overheating and made it easier to move the tip. The first two passes were performed with a long-pulse Nd:YAG laser. Patients then washed the face to remove gel residues, dried the skin, and cooled it with ice packs. One pass of the QS Nd:YAG (1064 nm) laser (Revlite, Cynosure, USA) was then performed. Each patient underwent a series of combined therapy sessions — a minimum of eight procedures. Initially, sessions were performed at 2–4 week intervals, which were subsequently lengthened depending on the response to therapy. In men, only QS Nd:YAG was used on facial hair growth areas to avoid the depilatory effects of the long-pulsed laser. Both lasers were used in other facial areas.

Parameters of long-pulsed Nd:YAG laser treatment:
- Wavelength: 1064 nm
- Spot size: 10 mm
- Pulse duration: 60 ms
- Energy density: 20–23 J/cm^2 depending on skin phototype

Parameters of QS Nd:YAG laser treatment:
- Wavelength: 1064 nm
- Spot size: 6 mm
- Energy density: 1.1–1.3 J/cm^2 also depending on a patient's skin type

Results. Initially, the severity of acne on a scale of 1 to 5 averaged points (range 2–5). All participating patients underwent 8–16 sessions (12 on average), and improvement was registered after 6–8 sessions.

Immediately after the final treatment session, the acne skin lesion area was reduced by 81% on average. At the same time, the skin condition of 45% of patients improved by 90%. Participants rated the overall improvement in appearance at 80%. At follow-up examinations, the achieved results were not only maintained but enhanced. The average reduction in acne-affected skin was 86%, and the improvement in appearance was achieved in 84% of the cases.

The only adverse effect was transient erythema, although all participants could return to their usual activities immediately after treatment. The procedures were very well tolerated — at their worst, the patient experienced only mild discomfort. Patients who used topical retinoids or oral antibiotics before or during laser treatment could theoretically have other complications. However, the evidence related to such adverse outcomes is scattered and sparse.

Thus, combined therapy with long-pulse and Q-switched (QS) Nd:YAG (1064 nm) lasers proved effective in treating moderate to severe acne. After the final session, the results persisted for almost two years without topical retinoids or oral antibiotics. This can be explained by the thermal effect on the pilosebaceous complex and reduction of *C. acnes*. In most cases, an improvement of follicular hyperkeratinization and suppression of cytokine-mediated inflammatory cascade was also noted, which probably plays a vital role in the initiation of skin lesions with acne (Kircik L.H., 2016).

Histological examination of areas exposed to Nd:YAG (1064 nm) laser radiation showed a decrease in inflammation with suppression of TLR-2, IL-8, NF-κB, TNF-α, and matrix metalloproteinase 9 (MMP-9) expression. This may explain the stable efficacy observed after combination therapy.

More information about laser and phototherapy can be found in the *Lasers in Cosmetic Dermatology & Skincare Practice* book.

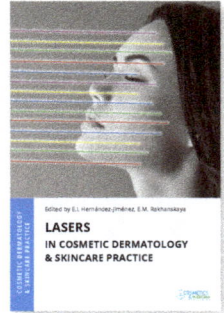

2.6.3. Drug therapy in combination with skincare and correction of the psychological status

Patient A., 18 years old, came to our clinic due to the presence of lesions on her chest and back (**Fig. IV-2-20**) insisting on oral isotretinoin prescription. She justified this request by the fact that her friend had been helped by isotretinoin. She further noted that, over the previous four years, she had already tried "many ointments" none of which yielded results. Her mood was low and anxious.

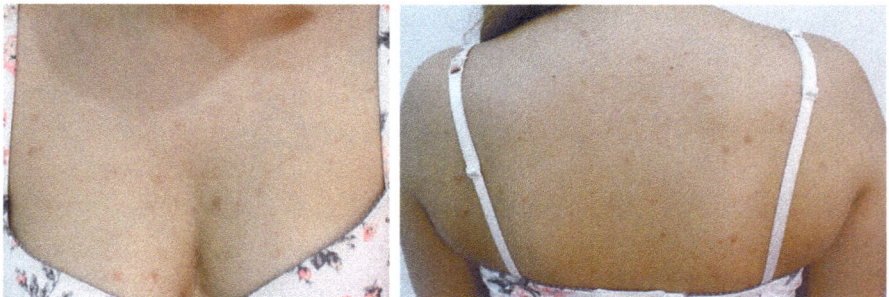

Figure IV-2-20. Patient A., 1st visit: signs of acne in the chest and back area (photo: Nikolaeva N.N.)

Medical history. The patient had been suffering from acne since she was 14 years old. Oily skin, blackheads, i.e., open and closed comedones in the T-zone of face, as well as the upper third of the chest and back, gradually became more prominent (exceeding the extent to which the same issues affected her mother at the same age). Later, patient claimed that sporadic papulopustular lesions formed, mainly on the chest and back.

She was worried about acne lesions and tried to disguise them with decorative cosmetics. She never sought help of a psychologist. She had no regular doctor to attend to her condition. She went to different dermatologists and aestheticians. Over the years, she used the following groups of medications that were recommended by doctors (according to the medical records provided by the patient):

- Benzoyl peroxide (applied it for two weeks, then stopped, as no effect)
- Topical antibacterial drugs with erythromycin (used for two months; she saw positive results at the beginning of therapy, but decided to discontinue their use because she was afraid that they contained antibiotics)
- Topical retinoids (redness and dryness of the skin appeared in a week, she was worried it would get worse and stopped)

In addition, the patient recalled relying on salicylic acid, calendula, hydrogen peroxide, chlorhexidine, and ichthyol ointment (these were the compounds she remembered). She chose these preparations on her own and used them haphazardly. She also used skincare cosmetics from various manufacturers, often simply applying soap and baby cream (when the skin was dry). Based on this experience, the patient concluded that external therapy would not help her.

Aesthetic history. The patient underwent mechanical cleansing several times but did not like that her face "turned red" after the treatment and redness persisted for 4–5 days, had one mesotherapy procedure (could not recall the name of the drug), had two fractional laser sessions one week apart (recalling that "it hurt, and it turned red again"). She also occasionally tried to perform manual cleaning by herself at home.

Gynecological history. First menstruation at age 13, the cycle was set immediately. An endocrinologist–gynecologist examination revealed no pathology.

Somatic status: no peculiarities.

Status localis. At the time of the examination, there were lesions on the face, back, and chest. On the face, there were post-inflammatory pigmentary spots and a few atrophic scars (the patient did not consent to having her face shown on photographs). Single papulopustular lesions were observed in the breast's upper third, and post-inflammatory pigmentary spots and atrophic scars were not pronounced. Lesions on the skin in the upper third of the back mostly manifested as post-inflammatory pigment spots and single papules.

Psycho-emotional status. According to the interview with the patient and test for determining the type of personality accentuation (TTPA), the patient can be characterized as an accentuated personality with a predominance of the anxious type of accentuation (**Fig. IV-2-21**). The bars (sensitivity, shyness, aggression, rigidity) on the chart, which go beyond the upper red line and indicate a deviation, are noteworthy.

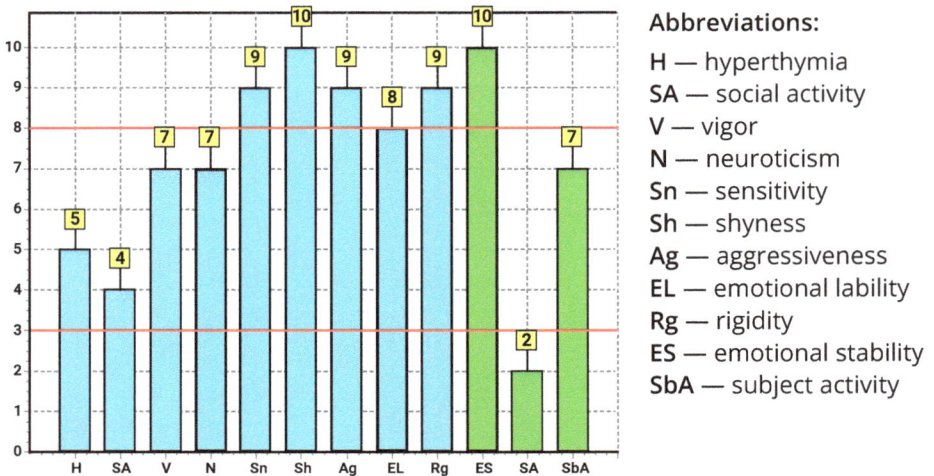

Abbreviations:
H — hyperthymia
SA — social activity
V — vigor
N — neuroticism
Sn — sensitivity
Sh — shyness
Ag — aggressiveness
EL — emotional lability
Rg — rigidity
ES — emotional stability
SbA — subject activity

Figure IV-2-21. Patient A., 1st visit: TTPA results

Women of this type are characterized by high sensitivity, emotional lability, low self-esteem, insecurity, and anxiety. Often, mood swings occur spontaneously, without any visible external reasons, and are accompanied by hyperexcitability of the vegetative nervous system, the experience of physical malaise, constant anxiety about their somatic condition, and the expression of vague somatic complaints. In these individuals, aggressive, angry reactions arise quickly, have an impulsive character, and are poorly controlled.

The personality features of this patient explain her attitude towards her illness (hypochondriacal) and treatment (expectation of quick results). Her inherent mood swings and fears prevented her from adhering to the rules she had been previously given for using external medications and care products. The patient's fidgetiness and anxiety can explain the chaotic use of topical drugs. Since the patient distrusts people, the absence of one attending physician is understandable.

Therapy. Considering the anamnesis data, objective examination (no indications for the prescription of isotretinoin), and the results of the psycho-emotional status assessment, the patient was recommended a course of external therapy in combination with psychological and aesthetic correction. The complex therapy included:

- Topical treatment to influence the pathological skin process: azelaic acid (cream 20%) on the lesions twice a day for four months
- Aesthetic treatment to improve skin quality: professional procedures with the use of surface peels and enzyme masks (10 sessions, four months)
- Psychological correction to remove emotional tension and form the motivation for treatment: conversations with elements of rational psychotherapy, relaxation sessions over a four-month period

Besides, considering the patient's experience of treatment (more precisely, her repeated violation of doctors' recommendations), the mechanism of action of azelaic acid, the purpose of prescription of this drug, time of clinical effect development, therapy duration, and the necessity of skincare was explained to the patient in detail. This reduced the patient's anxiety and several fears, and helped in the establishment of a trusting doctor–patient relationship. In addition, the patient's attention was drawn to the fact that it was necessary to observe the frequency and duration of treatment, which contributed to the patient's acceptance of personal responsibility for implementing recommendations and led to her optimistic attitude. As patients should believe in the results, making them understand their role in achieving the desired treatment effect is vital!

Results. The results of the comprehensive therapy are shown in **Fig. IV-2-22** and **Fig. IV-2-23** (all scales within the two red lines, no abnormalities). The patient was satisfied with her skin condition and noted that she was much calmer and had more plans, and that her quality of life had improved.

The described clinical case showed the effectiveness of external therapy for acne in combination with psychological correction, which in this case led to the patient's trust in the doctor, which improved her motivation to follow through with the treatment, as well as to establish a good attitude toward the disease and, correspondingly, to the administered medicines. This was an amazing achievement considering that the patient was initially against external therapy and asked the doctor to prescribe isotretinoin.

Thus, before abandoning external therapy and moving to systemic therapy, doctors should analyze the main factors of the ineffectiveness of external treatment in each case.

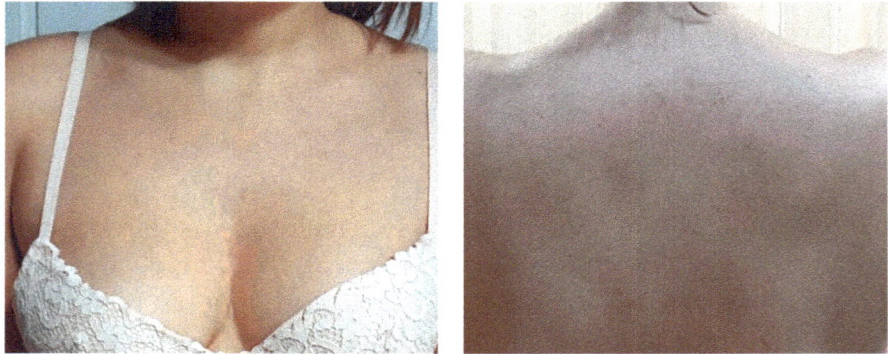

Figure IV-2-22. Patient A.: after therapy (photo: Nikolaeva N.N.)

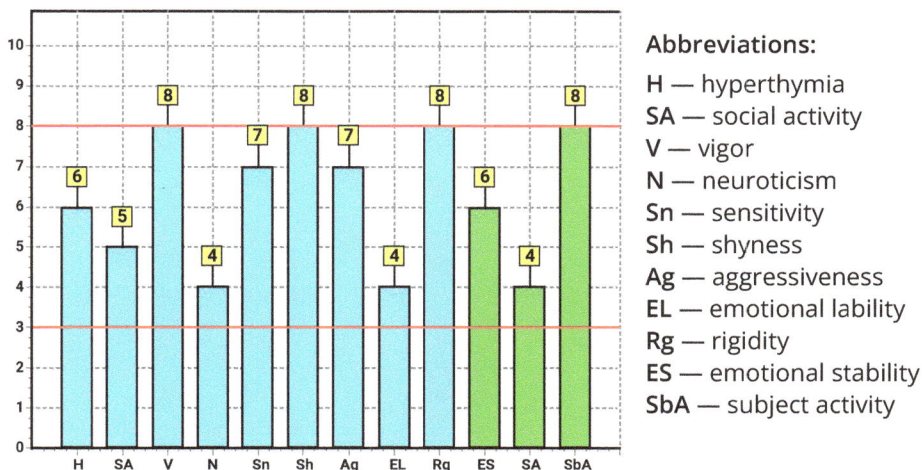

Abbreviations:
H — hyperthymia
SA — social activity
V — vigor
N — neuroticism
Sn — sensitivity
Sh — shyness
Ag — aggressiveness
EL — emotional lability
Rg — rigidity
ES — emotional stability
SbA — subject activity

Figure IV-2-23. Patient A.: TTPA results after therapy

We should not forget that trust (that the patient has in the doctor and vice versa) and cooperation (which requires that the doctor and the patient work in tandem) are essential components of the treatment process. Here, the words of Andrew Carnegie, an American entrepreneur, one of the world's wealthiest men, and the steel empire's founder, who donated 90% of his fortune to charity — come to mind: "There is no point in trying to help people who are not helping themselves. You can't make a man climb the ladder if he doesn't want to climb it himself."

Résumé

There is no monotherapy for acne (or a universal remedy). Therefore, the only valid and practical strategy is a comprehensive approach that includes:
1. Working with the skin with topical products and cosmetic procedures (regular manual cleansing in the first place!)
2. Protection of skin from harmful external influences (UV, air pollution, etc.)
3. Strengthening of general immunity (proper nutrition)
4. Improvement of psycho-emotional background

This protocol can be successfully implemented without the use of drugs, though not in 100% of cases. If the condition is acute and prolonged, medication will still need to be prescribed. In such cases, drug therapy should not be delayed unnecessarily; nonetheless, whenever possible, we should try to switch to skincare and aesthetic methods quickly.

Still, patients must accept that acne therapy is a long process the aim of which is to improve their condition without depleting their body's reserves.

Chapter 3
Post-acne

3.1. Symptoms and risk factors

Post-acne is a skin condition characterized by scars, enlarged pores, and pigmented spots. In some individuals, this triad remains for life after experiencing acne.

Although acne is widespread, patients do not always get to a specialist in time for diagnosis and treatment. Of all acne sufferers, only about 16% seek medical attention (Rivera A.E., 2008). Among them:

- 74% waited more than one year before seeing a physician
- 12% waited for 6 to 12 months
- 6% waited for 3 to 6 months
- Only 7% waited less than three months

These unfortunate statistics indicate that **educating patients and medical professionals is necessary because early and effective treatment can minimize the risk of post-inflammatory skin changes**.

In one study involving the histologic and immunologic investigation of the scarring process in acne, the following correlations were established:

1. When the inflammatory process is markedly active and resolves rapidly, the likelihood of scarring is lower than when the inflammatory response is mild and prolonged.
2. Lesions confined to the epidermis and papillary dermis can be repaired without forming scars. The outcome of this inflammatory process typically results in erythema and/or dyschromia. In contrast, the process located in the dermis tends to be more prolonged and can lead to the formation of hyper- or atrophic changes in the skin.

Another study, which involved 101 women and 84 men with varying numbers, morphology, and severity of acne on the face, chest, and back, showed that facial acne resulted in scarring of varying severity in 95% of participants of both genders. The obtained results further revealed that men are more prone to form hypertrophic and keloid scars (Rivera A.E., 2008).

Risk factors for scarring include:
- Severe inflammatory acne (although it can also occur with a mild form)
- Family history of acne
- Significant and prolonged inflammatory process
- Various manipulations of inflammatory lesions
- The appearance of acne at a young age
- Frequent relapses of the disease
- Localization in the trunk area

3.2. General approaches to post-acne prevention and treatment

3.2.1. Enlarged pores

Enlarged pores are associated with prolonged overstretching of the sebaceous ducts due to sebum accumulation. In addition, the quality of the dermal matrix changes with prolonged inflammation: its structural fibers become weaker, and its elasticity is impaired. The pores in these areas become even more overstretched as the resistance of the external tissue decreases (Lee S.J. et al., 2016).

The best prevention of apparent skin porosity is regular cleaning of the sebaceous gland ducts. If this is not done, glands will remain overstretched, even when their sebum production activity returns to normal. It is challenging to fight enlarged pores; even laser resurfacing does not give the desired effect. Nevertheless, some pore reduction is observed after procedures aimed at tightening the skin — microneedling, radiofrequency (RF)-lifting, fractional photo- and RF-thermolysis, IPL, and mesotherapy.

As for chemical peels and cosmetics, they have not proven themselves as post-acne scar corrective agents. This is not surprising, as they can be used to solve epidermal problems, which enlarged pores are not.

While the formation of enlarged pores is not directly related to inflammation, inflammation plays a significant role in the pathogenesis of the other two signs of post-acne — scarring and pigmentation disorders.

3.2.2. Post-acne scars

The inflammatory process undergoes three consecutive but overlapping stages — inflammation, granulation, and remodeling. If the basal membrane is involved, it ends in the formation of a normotrophic scar. When the balance of matrix metalloproteinases — MMP-1, -2, -9, and -13, proMMP-1 and -9, responsible for the architecture of the extracellular matrix, as well as their tissue inhibitors (TIMP) is disturbed, atrophic or hypertrophic scars form (Baranovsky Y.G. et al., 2016; Amirlak B. et al., 2017).

Another reason for the formation of post-acne scars may be peptidoglycan in the *C. acnes* cell wall, which, through the activation of proMMP-2 synthesis, enhances the degradation of the extracellular matrix (Baranovsky Y.G. et al., 2016; Amirlak B. et al., 2017).

Post-acne scars can be atrophic, hypertrophic, or keloid, with atrophic scars being three times more common on average.

Atrophic post-acne scars come in various shapes and sizes (Jacob C.I. et al., 2001). They can be V-shaped (icepick), M-shaped (rolling), or U-shaped (boxcar) (**Fig. IV-3-1** & **IV-3-2**).

- **V-shaped** scars are usually narrow (< 2 mm), sharply circumscribed, and can penetrate deep into the dermis or even into the subcutaneous tissue. These tissue defects are generally more comprehensive in the epidermis and become narrower as they deepen.
- **M-shaped** scars have a broad base (4–5 mm). These scars present as a wave-like structure of normal-looking skin. The undulations in the bottom of the scar are due to abnormal fibrous attachment of the dermis to the subcutaneous tissue.
- **U-shaped** scars present with a broader base than V-shaped scars but do not narrow. They appear as rounded or oval-shaped

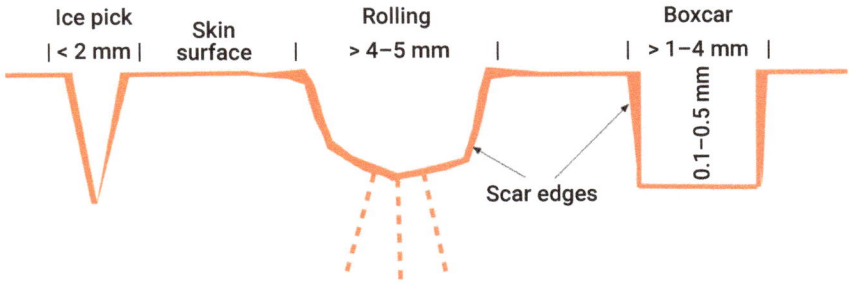

Figure IV-3-1. Shape of post-acne scars (adapted from Fabbrocini G. et al., 2010)

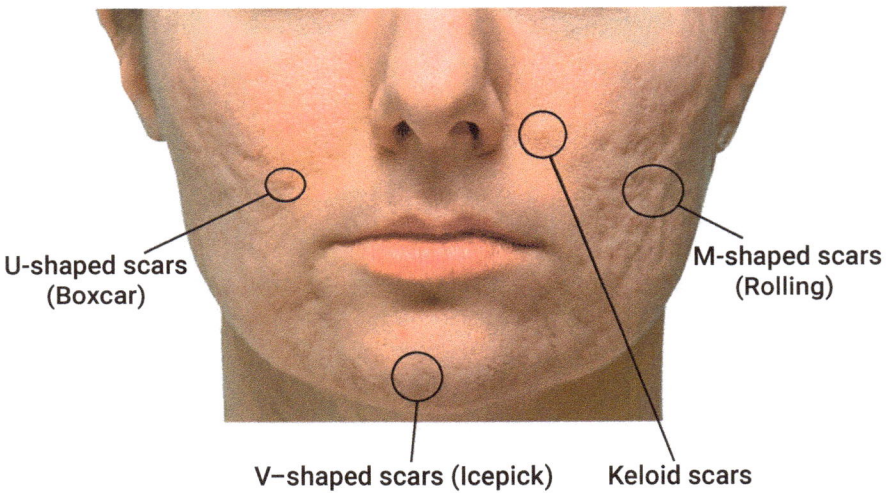

Figure IV-3-2. Types of post-acne scars

pits, have sharp edges, and can be either shallow (0.1–0.5 mm) or deep (>0.5 mm).

Hypertrophic scars rise above the skin's surface, forming lighter, denser areas within the trauma zone.

In contrast, **keloid** scars are soft, reddish–purple in color, and extend beyond the injured area.

Unfortunately, removing fully formed scars is impossible, but their severity can be significantly reduced. The choice of aesthetic method

Table IV-3-1. The post-acne scarring severity scale (Goodman G.J., Baron J.A., 2006)

DEGREE	CLINICAL MANIFESTATIONS
1 (macular)	Flat, erythematous, hyper- or hypopigmented lesions that do not disturb the skin topography
2 (mild)	Small atrophic or hypertrophic scars that are invisible from more than 0.5 m away. You can easily hide them with make-up or a beard (in men)
3 (moderate)	Atrophic or hypertrophic scars that are visible from more than 0.5 meters away. Not easily concealed by make-up or natural facial hair, but hardly visible when the skin is pulled taut
4 (severe)	Severe atrophic or hypertrophic scars are visible from a distance of more than 0.5 m. When the skin is pulled taut, the scars remain visible

is based on the scar severity. One of the classifications convenient for use in practice is given in **Table IV-3-1**.

Scarring occurs in severe acne when pustules extend deep into the dermis. Therefore, the earlier the work with acne begins (preferably while the acne is still in the noninflammatory stage), the lower the risk of scarring.

Post-acne scars are treated with fractional photo- or RF-thermolysis; the latter will be in the ablative procedure version using a micro-needle applicator. Some leveling of microrelief can be achieved with microdermabrasion, but the scars can cause a more profound damage than their primary effect.

3.2.3. Pigmentation and congestive spots

An equally common symptom of post-acne is secondary **hyper-pigmentation**. It can occur in patients with any skin phototype, especially in people with darker skin types and those who traumatize their inflammations. Dyschromias affect both men and women at any age with equal frequency. The color usually ranges from light brown to gray or black. Pigmentation becomes most prominent once inflammatory lesions and erythema disappear. Some researchers have observed that the heterogeneity of color often persists for a long time and brings more emotional discomfort than active forms of acne.

Secondary hyperpigmentation is due to the activation of melanogenesis at the site of inflammation. Melanocytes are stimulated by inflammatory mediators, cytokines, and arachidonic acid metabolites, increasing melanin synthesis and pigment deposition in the surrounding keratinocytes. Excessive melanin production and abnormal distribution lead to post-inflammatory pigmentation spots.

Hyperpigmentation is removed with lasers, chemical peeling, and cosmetic depigmentants.

Post-inflammatory **hypopigmentation** is rare but occurs in some cases (typically in the form of multiple small white spots in the scarring skin). Restoring the pigment in white depigmented areas is almost impossible. In this case, bleaching and lightening agents are recommended to lighten the pigmented areas slightly and make the white spots less contrasting. Make-up visually smooths out or even hides this aesthetic defect.

Congestive bluish spots on the skin are removed by improving microcirculation with the help of phototherapy (vascular laser, IPL), microcurrents, lymph drainage, temperature-based methods (RF heating and, conversely, cryomassage), and carboxytherapy.

Some methods for which the effectiveness has been proven through long-term clinical practice are discussed in more detail next.

3.3. Light therapy

3.3.1. Scar treatment

Laser therapy is the most general approach to post-acne scar reduction. The choice of laser device and parameters is determined by the scar type and affected area. To identify atrophic regions more accurately, it is advisable to illuminate the skin well during examination. Using a mirror to identify the most problematic areas with the patient is also recommended. Assessment of the physical characteristics of the scar (color, depth, width, depth) and its manifestation during skin stretching is critical (**Table IV-3-2**; **Fig. IV-3-3** & **IV-3-4**).

Table IV-3-2. Lasers for treating post-acne scars: tasks & devices

TASK	DEVICE
Skin resurfacing and remodeling (solid laser beam)	Ablative: • Carbon dioxide laser (CO_2, 10,600 nm) • Erbium laser (Er:YAG, 2940 nm)
Skin remodeling, stimulation of neocollagenesis, restoration of epidermis and dermis (fractional lasers)	Non-ablative: • Neodymium laser (Nd:YAG, 1320 nm) • Diode laser (1450 nm), • Erbium on glass laser (Er:glass, 1540 nm) • Thulium laser (1927 nm) Ablative: • Carbon dioxide laser (CO_2, 10,600 nm) • Erbium laser (Er:YAG, 2940 nm) • Spatially modulated ablation (Er:YAG/SMA, 2940 nm)
Vascular coagulation	• Pulsed dye laser (PDL, 585–595 nm) • Intense pulsed light device (IPL, 500–1200 nm) • Potassium titanyl phosphate crystal laser (KTP, 532, 1079/540 nm) • Neodymium laser (Nd:YAG, 1064 nm)

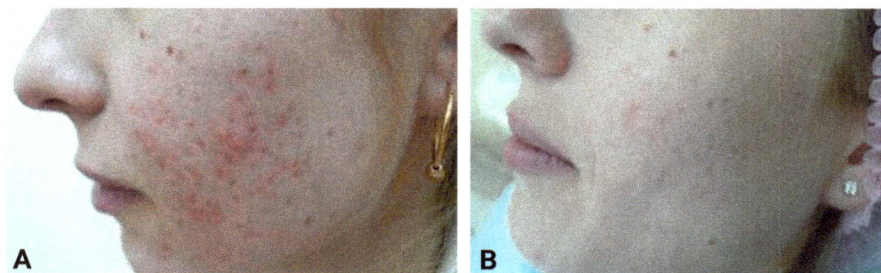

Figure IV-3-3. Post-acne: A — before treatment; B — four months after four sessions of QS Nd:YAG/KTP (1079/540 nm) with two-week intervals between procedures (photo: Urakova D.S., Kalashnikova N.G.)

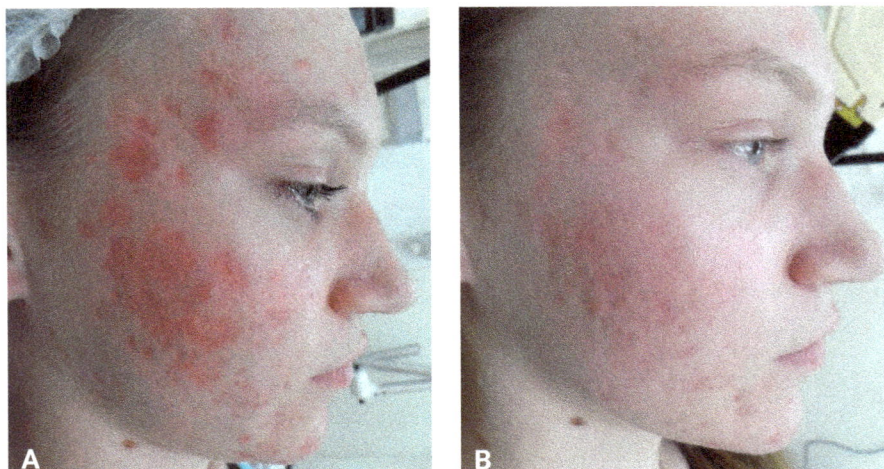

Figure IV-3-4. Moderate acne: A — before treatment; B — four months after therapy (QS Nd:YAG (1079 nm) — two sessions with a two-week interval; QS Nd:YAG/KTP (1079/540 nm) — two sessions; Er:YAG/SMA — one session) (photo: Urakova D.S., Kalashnikova N.G.)

Atrophic scars

There are many methods for atrophic scar treatment. Often their combination leads to better results than monotherapy. Such a combination allows for the destruction of the defective tissue and activates the remodeling and restoration of the epidermis and dermis. Unfortunately, no therapy removes these scars entirely.

Atrophic scars can be remodeled with fractional ablative and nonablative lasers. Fractional photothermolysis differs from laser resurfacing, which completely removes the surface layer of the skin, leaving wounds. In contrast, fractional photothermolysis creates columns of thermal damage down to the deep layers in the dermis, resembling "pixels in a photo." The epidermis around such thermal injury columns heals quickly, significantly reducing the recovery time.

To improve the appearance of the skin, the scar is resurfaced with a continuous beam of CO_2 (10,600 nm) or Er:YAG (2940 nm) laser radiation. Ablative laser remodeling aims to vaporize moisture-containing skin structures to the papillary dermis. Although the ablation depth is directly related to the number of passes performed, it is usually limited to the epidermis and the papillary dermis.

Radiation from pulsed Er:YAG lasers is ten times better absorbed by water than CO_2 laser radiation. Hence, their use results in better tissue evaporation and reduced residual thermal damage to the dermis. Thus, short-pulse Er:YAG laser resurfacing in several passes allows high-quality removal of the superficial layers of defective tissue. However, because it is accompanied only by ablation and no zone of adjacent thermal damage, it provides less collagen shrinkage than observed during treatment with a CO_2 laser. Therefore, for a milder degree of atrophic scarring, Er:YAG may be the preferred method, given the shorter postoperative recovery time, as confirmed by the histological pattern obtained in a study performed on small laboratory animals. Φlmost complete epithelialisation was observed on Day 10 visually and histologically (**Fig. IV-3-5**).

M- and U-shaped scars can be remodeled with laser ablation. On the other hand, V-shaped and U-shaped deep scars should not be subjected to total ablation and should instead be treated with fractional photothermolysis. For example, according to some reports, atrophic pigmented scars on swarthy skin can be successfully treated with a fractional CO_2 laser (Arsiwala S.Z., Desai S.R., 2019).

Non-ablative lasers generate light in the infrared range of electromagnetic radiation (1000–1500 nm). Such radiation has a lower water absorption coefficient, penetrating deeper tissues without causing ablation (only coagulation), leaving the *stratum corneum* intact.

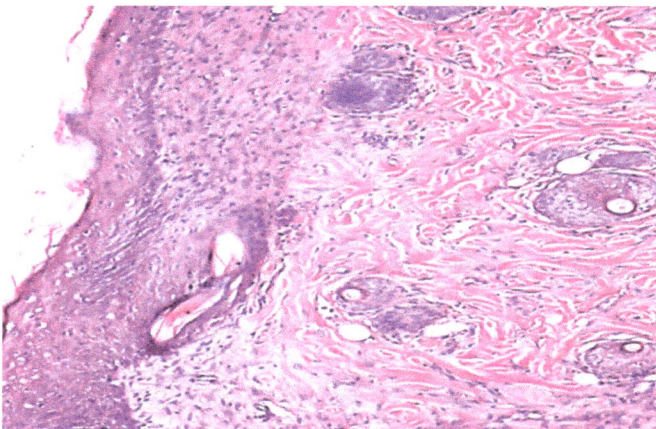

Figure IV-3-5. Histological picture on Day 10 after treatment with Er:YAG (staining with hematoxylin and eosin 100×)

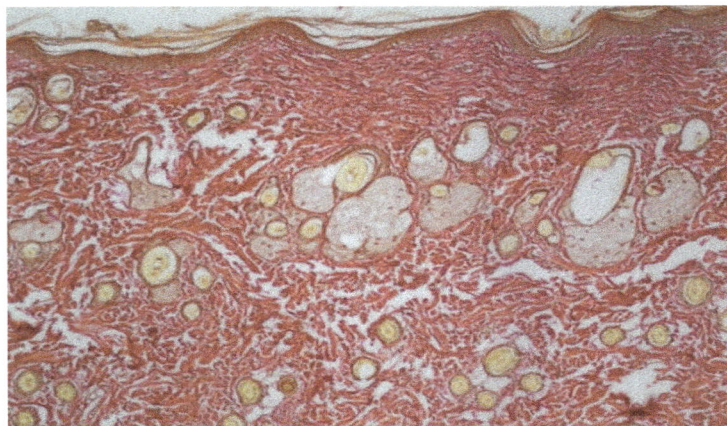

Figure IV-3-6. Histological picture on Day 10 after treatment with Er:YAG/SMA (staining with hematoxylin and eosin 100×)

This mechanism of skin injury stimulates the formation of new collagen and elastin, which improves post-acne appearance. In one of our cases, skin histology on the 10th day after exposure to Er:YAG/SMA showed staining of collagen fibers, which had varying degrees of intensity and indicated different degrees of connective tissue maturity (neocollagenogenesis), while preserving pronounced blood supply and angiogenesis (**Fig. IV-3-6**) (Urakova D.S., Kalashnikova N.G., 2015).

Regardless of the device used, the following objectives are pursued during atrophic scar treatment:

1. Leveling the border between the atrophic and the intact (normal) skin surrounding the scar
2. Stimulating collagen production in the atrophic area

Hypertrophic and keloid scars

Hypertrophic and keloid scars form due to abnormal inflammatory processes and healing, leading to tissue overgrowth because of insufficient MMP activity. There is persistent and intense local inflammation at the injury site with the involvement of inflammatory cells and fibroblasts, forming new blood vessels and collagen — together, they form a scar.

Hypertrophic scars are limited to the inflammation area. These scars persist during the first two months after the injury and tend to normal maturation and regression of hypertrophic masses, unlike keloids.

Typically, they are localized in the region of the lateral surfaces of the face, the chin and neck, and the upper part of the trunk.

Combining several laser methods is recommended for treating this type of scar. In addition to removing abnormal tissue and activating remodeling by the procedures mentioned above, the vascular component of the scar is also targeted for vessel coagulation.

Laser treatment of the vessels is based on the theory of selective photothermolysis proposed by Richard Rox Anderson and John Parrish. According to this perspective, specific skin molecules — chromophores — actively absorb certain types of radiation. Suppose the energy of laser radiation with a particular wavelength is transferred to the chromophore for a time that is shorter than its thermal relaxation time (TRT). In that case, it is possible to damage the target without involving the surrounding tissues that do not contain the chromophore. Consequently, the laser must emit electromagnetic waves with a specific wavelength absorbed by the target chromophore. The primary chromophore in blood vessels is hemoglobin. After absorption, the light energy is converted into heat, which leads to the coagulation of hemoglobin, erythrocytes, and vessel walls. The final stage of aseptic inflammation will be thrombosis and vessel occlusion.

Various types of vascular lasers and broadband light sources are used for this purpose:

- Pulsed dye laser (PDL, 585–595 nm)
- Intense pulsed light (IPL, 500–1200 nm)
- Potassium titanyl phosphate crystal laser (KTP, 532, 1079/540 nm)
- Neodymium laser (Nd:YAG, 1064 nm)

Although it is recommended to combine vascular lasers with fractional photothermolysis, the sole use of the former can provide improvement in scar tissue.

There is no consensus on how vascular lasers, particularly PDL (the most investigated type of vascular laser), provide clinical improvement in scar therapy. Laser-induced damage to the microcirculatory bed is assumed to lead to tissue hypoxia followed by collagen degradation through collagenase release. Further thermal damage of collagen fibers leads to dissociation of disulfide bonds and their rearrangement and an increase in the number of regional mast cells, which can stimulate collagen (Amirlak B. et al., 2017). After removing the vascular component in the scar and inducing changes in its characteristics, it is possible to proceed to fractional photothermolysis.

3.3.2. Post-acne pigmentation

The following laser and broadband light sources can be used to remove post-inflammatory pigmentation:
- Pulsed dye laser (PDL, 585–595 nm)
- Frequency-doubled neodymium laser (QS Nd:YAG/KTP, 1064/532, 1079/540 nm)
- Frequency-doubled ruby laser (QS Ruby, 694 nm)
- Frequency-doubled alexandrite laser (QS Alexandrite, 755 nm)
- Frequency-doubled neodymium laser (QS Nd:YAG, 1064 nm)

Laser treatment of pigmented lesions is also based on the theory of selective photothermolysis. The spectrum band where the best radiation absorption by melanin is observed lies between 630 and 1100 nm and is called the **melanin window** (Rahanskaya E.M., 2016). Melanin absorption decreases as the radiation wavelength increases, but laser light of longer wavelengths penetrates deeper into the skin.

Pulsed light sources, unlike lasers, generate light across the entire emitted spectrum (400 to 1200 nm). Therefore, this radiation affects not only melanin but also hemoglobin, collagen, and water, which can even out skin tone and slightly improve its structure. Still, if needed, the radiation parameters of IPL devices can be adjusted with special spectral filters.

In addition to pigment lasers and IPLs, ablative and non-ablative fractional photothermolysis can also be used to treat hyperpigmentation. As a result of the energy absorbed by the water molecules of living skin cells, melanocytes are also damaged. After fractional exposure, microepidermal necrotic debris is formed in the tissue, containing cell fragments, destroyed collagen and elastin fibers, and large amounts of melanin. After the recovery period, the skin takes on an even shade.

When treating post-inflammatory hyperpigmentation, one should not forget the risk of secondary stimulation of melanin production. Prevention of this type of complication requires appropriately chosen radiation parameters and strict observance of specialist recommendations.

3.3.3. Post-procedure recommendations

Patients undergoing laser therapy should abide by the following rules:
- Avoid sunbathing for at least two weeks or until the skin has fully recovered if the procedure was accompanied by skin damage
- Use topical products that normalize the wound healing process
- Use sunscreens with sun protection factor (SPF) 50
- Do not traumatize the treatment area
- Topical preparations should be avoided 2–3 days before and after the procedure
- Laser treatment is possible only four months after discontinuing the use of systemic retinoids and seven days after completing the the photosensitizing drug therapy

3.4. RF therapy

Radiofrequency (RF) therapy's active factor is a high-frequency alternating electric current (4–6 MHz) generated in the skin by its contact with electrodes to which alternating voltage is applied. This type of electric current heats the skin. The degree of heating and the depth where the temperature rises to the maximum depends on the electrodes' shape and the modes of voltage application to them. It is essential to note that the focus of heating can be profound while the surface itself will be minimally heated.

The electrodes can be placed on the skin surface (pin electrodes) or can be used to pierce the skin (needle electrodes). Fractional RF is best suited for post-acne treatment. It is delivered via applicators with multiple electrodes — pins (which have a small area of contact with the skin, but it is not pierced) or needles.

As a result, microscopic zones of thermal ablation and coagulation are created in the dermis. With pin electrodes, there is no damage to the epidermis and the *stratum corneum*. That is why this technique is called non-ablative. This is a gentler treatment; it is less painful and does not require a rehabilitation period. After a series of non-ablative procedures, there is a tightening of the skin associated with some narrowing of the pores. But for scars, such an effect is not enough.

Ablative fractional RF technology is used with needle applicators to loosen the scar tissue and stimulate reparation. Microneedling RF has a dual action: on the one hand, it directly damages the skin, triggering reparation in the epidermis and dermis; on the other hand, it heats the skin, activating cellular and tissue metabolism.

An exciting study exploring the potential of this technology was published in 2019 in the Journal of Drugs in Dermatology (Katz B., 2019). It involved 15 patients of Fitzpatrick skin phototypes II–VI with post-acne scars and inflammatory lesions. Each patient underwent three facial treatments at 3–4 week intervals (according to individual skin condition and physician's decision)

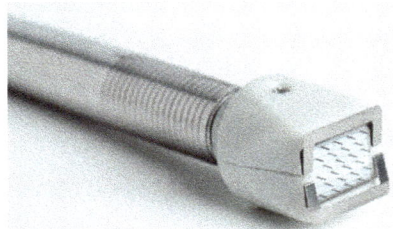

Figure IV-3-7. Fractora handpiece with 24-pin tip (InMode, Israel)

using an applicator with 24 needle electrodes of 2500 μm length each (**Fig. IV-3-7**) with or without 2000 μm of insulating coating. The applicator with insulated needles was used at the physician's discretion for dark skin types. The safety and efficacy of the therapy were evaluated at three follow-up visits: 1, 3, and 6 months after the last treatment.

Skin reactions in the form of erythema and mild to moderate edema, spot bleeding, and acne exacerbation were transient and resolved spontaneously without any intervention. However, with each subsequent visit, there was a gradual improvement in the skin condition compared with the initial one. Thus, the post-acne scar severity score decreased from an average of 2.80 to 0.80, the inflammatory lesions from 2.93 to 0.75, and the overall skin condition improved from 1.45 points after one treatment to 3.50 points six months after treatment (**Fig. IV-3-8**).

In contrast to previous studies (Taub A.F., Garretson C.B., 2011; Elman M. et al., 2012; Chandrashekar B.S. et al., 2014; Harth Y. et al., 2014; Hellman J., 2016; Hellman J., Yao J., 2019), this study is notable because it involved patients who had acne that had not resolved. Yet, the therapy did not cause any significant or unexpected adverse reactions. The improvement manifested not only in the assessment of post-acne scars but also in acne lesions and overall skin condition.

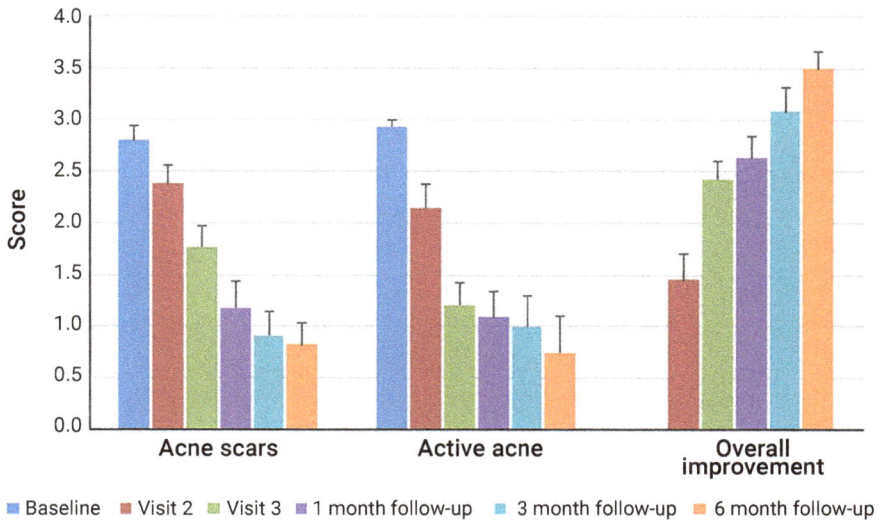

Figure IV-3-8. Score changes reflecting the severity of post-acne, active acne, and the appearance of the skin during the treatment and after one, three, and six months of observation compared with the initial state

The improvement was gradual because collagen and elastin regeneration and, consequently, skin renewal is a process that takes time.

As for pigmentation, after RF microneedling, there is observed evening of skin tone because of scaling. However, this method cannot effectively treat post-inflammatory pigmentation.

3.5. Microneedling

Microneedling is a popular procedure for treating aesthetic skin problems localized in the dermal layer. These are deep wrinkles, atrophic post-burn, post-traumatic or post-acne scars, as well as pigmentation disorders such as melasma and post-inflammatory hyperpigmentation at the edges of the scar, where the pigment can be found in the dermal layer (Fabbrocini G. et al., 2009; Alam M. et al., 2014).

Microneedling creates multiple punctures in the skin by applying a roller the surface of which is dotted with many needles of 0.25–1.5 mm diameter (this device is called a mesoroller or dermaroller). Trauma triggers reparative processes in the skin, which ideally should lead to the replacement of malformed structures with normal ones. Trauma during microneedling is always full-layer and involves the epidermis and dermis (even in the case of short needles) (Kravvas G., Al-Niaimi F., 2017).

Unlike fractional RF, which traumatizes and warms the skin at depth without superficial burns, microneedling has only one active factor — mechanical trauma (El-Domyati M. et al., 2015, 2018). To expand the therapeutic possibilities of microneedling, it is combined with topical solutions of active substances. For example, a vitamin C solution followed by meso-roller treatment is recommended to improve skin texture (skin thickening and pore narrowing) and lighten pigmentation. Pre-application of platelet-rich plasma to the skin enhances the overall condition and appearance of the skin (Chawla S., 2014). There are reports of a successful combination of microneedling and glycolic peel in post-acne therapy (Sharad J., 2011). In general, such a combination is justified — the effect of microneedling is mainly related to the reorganization of the dermal matrix, and glycolic peel solves epidermal problems (pigmentation and keratosis).

3.6. Dermabrasion and microdermabrasion

Dermabrasion involves consistent resurfacing of the skin with abrasive materials that separate the upper layers of the epidermis: the smaller the abrasive particles, the less damage the procedure will cause. Dermabrasion to the basal membrane is painful and requires long rehabilitation. Today this method is rarely used in practice since there are safer and more effective alternatives for solving dermal problems. But microdermabrasion, which works within the *stratum corneum*, is very popular. There are two primary varieties of microdermabrasion.

1. **Crystal microdermabrasion** is performed by treating the skin surface with a jet of microcrystalline powder. In most cases, aluminum oxide is used, but there are devices using microcrystals of magnesium oxide, sodium bicarbonate (soda), and sodium chloride (table salt). Mechanical removal of skin flakes opens pores and triggers the cell turnover in the epidermis, while jet application reflexively stimulates microcirculation of deep skin layers.

2. **Diamond microdermabrasion** is carried out using rotating nozzles with diamond coating and vacuum suction, gently re-

moving the keratinized surface skin layers. This superficial procedure can be performed on the face, neck, décolletage, and other body parts, irrespective of the skin type.

Microdermabrasion solves epidermal problems such as keratosis and hyperpigmentation. With this method, it is impossible to remove scars, although it is possible to improve their appearance by smoothing the skin's relief (El-Domyati M. et al., 2016).

Since microdermabrasion damages the *stratum corneum* over a large area, after the procedure, the skin must be particularly carefully protected until the *stratum corneum* is restored. For this purpose, special wound-healing topical products on an emulsion (or even ointment) basis with occlusive properties are used. Gel-based preparations are unsuitable because they quickly evaporate water, and the treated skin area, unable to retain water on its own, will become moisture deficient.

3.7. Dermal fillers

Dermal fillers are used to even out the skin relief and make atrophic scars less noticeable. There are publications in the medical literature describing the use of different materials:

- Polylactic acid (Sapra S. et al., 2015)
- Hyaluronic acid (Artzi O. et al., 2020)
- Polymethacrylate (Joseph J.H., 2019)
- Collagen (Sage R.J. et al., 2011)
- Calcium hydroxyapatite (Koren A., 2019)

Most of these publications provide descriptions of clinical cases from the authors' practice, although there are also some literature reviews (De Boulle K., Heydenrych I., 2015; Wollina U., Goldman A., 2015).

There is no specificity in the choice of material and technique of injection when working with post-acne scars; here, we should be guided by indications and contraindications for a particular filler. The only recommendation is to prefer biodegradable fillers with a proven high safety profile.

Hyaluronic fillers give a quick volumizing effect. They degrade over time and have a stimulatory impact on fibroblasts, promoting the synthesis of new extracellular matrix components, mainly mucopolysaccharides. As for collagen and hydroxyapatite, these materials have poorly expressed volumetric effects but activate the production of collagen and elastin structural fibers. Thus, while we can assume the clinical impact of using volumetric and stimulating fillers, this expected effect must be checked for safety via histological studies since there is a general recommendation not to use fillers of varying chemical groups in one area of the skin.

In this regard, combining physical remodeling techniques with volumetric filler injections, avoiding possible "conflicts" among methods, is advised (Biesman B.S. et al., 2019). However, even here, the issue of protocols remains open.

3.8. Mesotherapy, biorevitalization, carboxytherapy

Intradermal injections of different bioactive substances can influence various physiological processes.

Mesosolutions with antioxidants (primarily vitamin C) and synthetic peptides regulating melanin production are mainly indicated for pigment lesions. To promptly supply the skin with necessary building substances, dermal injections of amino acids and nucleotides in combination with fractional physical methods are recommended.

High-molecular-weight native hyaluronic acid used for skin biorevitalization helps tighten the skin and narrow the pores.

Carboxytherapy, the intradermal injection of carbon dioxide, improves skin metabolism. The action of this method is based on the acidification of the intercellular fluid. Upon dissolving in water, carbon dioxide forms carbonic acid and lowers the pH value. This leads to an expansion of capillaries and increases blood flow to the treatment area. As a result, the metabolic and respiratory processes in the cells are activated, which will have a general healing effect on the skin.

3.9. Chemical peeling

According to modern concepts, chemical peeling is an aesthetic treatment for solving primarily epidermal problems. Phenol and TCA, used for many years for deep peeling, are now prohibited for safety reasons. They are highly toxic substances, and their health risks are entirely unwarranted, especially since new aesthetic technologies allow for effective and safe work at the dermal level.

The roughness of the post-acne skin is associated with an uneven *stratum corneum*. In the scar area, it is usually thinner, while in the neighboring regions, it is thickened. When treating hyperkeratosis, salicylic or Jessner peeling is the best. Still, for gradual smoothing and softening of the *stratum corneum*, preference should be given to enzymatic or superficial acid peeling (in addition to glycolic acid, almond, pyruvic, and lactic acids are desirable) (Garg V.K. et al., 2009; Sachdeva S., 2010).

Retinol and acid peels should be used to even out tone and lighten pigment spots (Chandrashekar B.S. et al., 2015).

As for enlarged pores and scarring, chemical peeling (even a medium-depth!) cannot solve these problems. In some cases, there may be some improvement in the appearance of scars. However, it is not comparable with the effect of fractional laser, RF, or microneedling.

3.10. Cosmetic products

People with post-acne do not necessarily have oily skin. Moreover, over time, they may experience a lack of sebum. Measurements often show a decrease in the *stratum corneum* hydration and an increase in the transepidermal water loss index (TEWL). This indicates that the *stratum corneum* does not hold water properly, and its barrier function has weakened.

Here are a few rules to follow when choosing cosmetics for post-acne.

1. **The first point of reference is the level of sebum production.** If it is decreased, preference should be given to products for dry low-sebum skin; for example, products for cleansing and care of atopic and xerotic skin. If there is too much sebum, products for oily skin should be used (see Part IV, section 1.2).
2. **Use depigmenting cosmetics with caution.** Depigmenting substances that inhibit melanogenesis can irritate the skin. Therefore, their prolonged use should be avoided. Preference should be given to superficial peels with a lightning effect. Depigmentants must be applied spot-on, not all over the face.
3. **Antioxidants are beneficial for post-acne skin.** Thanks to their anti-inflammatory properties, antioxidants will be effective in

the prevention of the darkening of existing pigment lesions and the appearance of new ones. In this regard, you should pay special attention to highly concentrated vitamin C. Vitamin C can be in pure form as a dried powder, which must be diluted in water before applying it to the skin, or in gel form (so-called serums). In antioxidant serums, vitamin C can be combined with other antioxidant substances, e.g., vitamin E and ferulic acid. Vitamin C antioxidant serums can be used with microneedling (see Part IV, section 3.4).

4. **Products with vitamin A (retinol)** can be chosen from anti-age cosmetic lines considering the patient's level of skin oiliness. In preparations for low-sebum skin, the total concentration of the retinol and retinol derivatives is lower than in those for oily skin.

5. **Do not use alcohol lotions with astringent agents.** Alcohol (especially in products containing acetone) further weakens the already weak barrier of post-acne skin and dries out the *stratum corneum*. Astringent substances are tannins, a group of phenolic substances of plant origin containing many –OH groups. The tanning effect is based on tannin's ability to form chemical bonds with proteins, polysaccharides, and other biopolymers. These substances are conventionally used for treating leather and fur, and for textile fiber etching. But in the case of live skin, their frequent use leads to drying of the *stratum corneum* and deterioration of its barrier function. Yes, tannins visually narrow pores, but this narrowing is temporary and occurs due to changes in the *stratum corneum* at the sebaceous gland's orifice; deep down in the skin, the pores are still dilated. So, such products do not solve the problem of enlarged pores but undermine the skin's barrier function.

6. **Photoprotection is necessary for post-acne skin.** When choosing the product, two things should be considered: (1) the UV radiation level and (2) the activity of sebum production. SPF value should be selected according to the actual solar activity in the patient's region. If sunscreens with unreasonably high SPF are used, there is a risk of affecting the physiological production of vitamin D in the skin. A choice of the cosmetic product form is based on the level of sebum: for low-sebum skin, a denser base (emulsion or even oil) should be chosen; for oily skin, it is a light emulsion or gel emulsion.

Résumé

Post-acne is a dermatologic condition involving epidermal and dermal problems, so post-acne treatment must involve a combination of aesthetic methods (**Table IV-3-3**). Their use in the therapy framework must be based on an in-depth understanding of the mechanisms of action, clinical effects, and contraindications. In our book, we have tried to give a brief but comprehensive explanation of when and why a particular method may be helpful.

In conclusion, once again, note the critical importance of preventive work — it must begin in the earliest stages manifesting in the appearance of the first signs of increased sebum production. Proper skincare for oily skin can prevent or significantly reduce the severity of acne and its consequences.

Table IV-3-3. Aesthetic methods for post-acne treatment

TOOLS & METHODS	EPIDERMAL PROBLEMS			DERMAL PROBLEMS	
	KERA-TOSIS	WEAKENED BARRIER	PIGMEN-TATION	ENLARGED PORES	SCARS
Light technology	+	–	+++	+	+++
RF technology	+	–	+	+	+++
Microneedling	+	–	–	+	++
Dermal fillers	–	–	–	–	++
Biorevitalization	–	–	–	+	+
Mesotherapapy	–	–	+	+	+
Injectable carboxytherapy	+	+	–	–	+
Dermabrasion/ microdermabrasion	+++	–	+	–	–
Chemical peeling	++	–	+++	–	–
Cosmetic products	++	+++	++	–	–

"–" — no effect; "+" — weak effect; "++" — moderate effect; "+++" — the most pronounced effect

References

Aktaş Karabay E., Aksu Çerman A. Demodex folliculorum infestations in common facial dermatoses: acne vulgaris, rosacea, seborrheic dermatitis. An Bras Dermatol 2020; 95(2): 187–193.

Alam M., Han S., Pongprutthipan M. et al. Efficacy of a needling device for the treatment of acne scars: a randomized clinical trial. JAMA Dermatol 2014; 150: 844–849.

Alcolea J.M., Hernández E., Martínez-Carpio P.A. et al. Treatment of chronic lower extremity ulcers with a new Er:YAG laser technology. Laser Therapy 2014; 23(6): 211–222.

Amirlak B., Unger J.G., Kenkel J.M. Laser treatment of scars and stria distensae. Medscape 2017; https://emedicine.medscape.com/article/1120673-overview?form=fpf.

Arora M.K., Yadav A., Saini V. Role of hormones in acne vulgaris. Clin Biochem 2011; 44: 1035–1040.

Arsiwala S.Z., Desai S.R. Fractional carbon dioxide laser: optimizing treatment outcomes for pigmented atrophic acne scars in skin of color. J Cutan Aesthet Surg 2019; 12(2): 85–94.

Artzi O., Cohen S., Koren A. et al. Dual-plane hyaluronic acid treatment for atrophic acne scars. J Cosmet Dermatol 2020; 19(1): 69–74.

Bagatin E., dos Santos Guadanhim L.R., Yarak S. et al. Dermabrasion for acne scars during treatment with oral isotretinoin. Dermatol Surg 2010; 36: 483–489.

Bakus A.D., Yaghmai D., Massa M.C. et al. Sustained benefit after treatment of acne vulgaris using only a novel combination of long-pulsed and Q-Switched 1064-nm Nd:YAG lasers. Dermatol Surg 2018; 44(11): 1402–1410.

Balak D.M.W. Topical trifarotene: a new retinoid. Br J Dermatol 2018; 179(2): 231–232.

Balić A., Vlašić D., Žužul K. et al. Omega-3 versus omega-6 polyunsaturated fatty acids in the prevention and treatment of inflammatory skin diseases. Int J Mol Sci 2020; 21(3): 741.

Baranovsky Y.G., Ilchenko F.N., Shapovalova E.Y., Artemov Y.V. Apoptotic and proliferative cell activity of pathological scars. Bull Emergency Reconstr Surg 2016; 3(1): 379–383.

Barrault C., Garnier J., Pedretti N. et al. Androgens induce sebaceous differentiation in sebocyte cells expressing a stable functional andro-gen receptor. J Steroid Biochem Mol Biol 2015; 152: 34–44.

Biesman B.S., Cohen J.L., DiBernardo B.E. et al. Treatment of atrophic facial acne scars with microneedling followed by polymethylmethacrylate-collagen gel dermal filler. Dermatol Surg 2019; 45(12): 1570–1579.

Birkmeyer G.J., Lazuk A.V. Restoration of cellular energy with NADH drugs in the prevention and treatment of chronic fatigue syndrome. Cosmetics and Medicine 2018; 3: 80–87.

Borrel V., Thomas P., Catovic C. et al. Acne and stress: impact of catecholamines on cutibacterium acnes. Front Med (Lausanne) 2019; 6: 155.

Casas M.N., Monaco M., Magliano J., Bazzano C. Hard-to-diagnose unilateral facial dermatosis. Clin Case Rep J 2020; 1(5): 1–3.

Chandrashekar B.S., Ashwini K.R., Vasanth V. et al. Retinoic acid and glycolic acid combination in the treatment of acne scars. Indian Dermatol Online J 2015; 6: 84–88.

Chandrashekar B.S., Sriram R., Mysore R. et al. Evaluation of microneedling fractional radio-frequency device for treatment of acne scars. J Cutan Aesthet Surg 2014; 7: 93–97.

Chawla S. Split face comparative study of microneedling with PRP versus microneedling with vitamin C in treating atrophic post acne scars. J Cutan Aesthet Surg 2014; 7: 209–212.

Chugunov A. Antihistamines regulate sebaceous gland activity. a new perspective on antihistamine therapy in the treatment of acne. Peelings 2011; 2: 40–45.

Clayton R.W., Langan E.A., Ansell D.M. et al. Neuroendocrinology and neurobiology of sebaceous glands. Biol Rev Camb Philos Soc 2020; 95(3): 592–624.

Contassot E., Beer H.D., French L.E. Interleukin-1, inflammasomes, autoinflammation and the skin. Swiss Med Wkly 2012; 142: 13590.

Darne S., Hiscutt E.L., Seukeran D.C. Evaluation of the clinical efficacy of the 1,450 nm laser in acne vulgaris: a randomized split-face, investigator-blinded clinical trial. Br J Dermatol 2011; 165: 1256–1262.

De Boulle K., Heydenrych I. Patient factors influencing dermal filler complications: Prevention, assessment, and treatment. Clin Cosmet Investig Dermatol 2015; 8: 205–214.

Dogan G. Possible isotretinoin-induced keloids in a patient with Behcet's disease. Clin Exp Dermatol 2006; 31: 535–537.

Dréno B., Pécastaings S., Corvec S. et al. Cutibacterium acnes (Propionibacterium acnes) and acne vulgaris: a brief look at the latest updates. J Eur Acad Dermatol Venereol 2018; 32(Suppl 2): 5–14.

El-Domyati M., Abdel-Wahab H., Hossam A. Microneedling combined with platelet-rich plasma or trichloroacetic acid peeling for management of acne scarring: a split-face clinical and histologic comparison. J Cosmet Dermatol 2018; 17(1): 73–83.

El-Domyati M., Barakat M., Awad S. et al. Microneedling therapy for atrophic acne scars: An objective evaluation. J Clin Aesthet Dermatol 2015; 8: 36–42.

El-Domyati M., Hosam W., Abdel-Azim E. et al. Microdermabrasion: a clinical, histometric, and histopathologic study. J Cosmet Dermatol 2016; 15: 503–513.

Ellis S.R., Nguyen M., Vaughn A.R. et al. The skin and gut microbiome and its role in common dermatologic conditions. Microorganisms 2019; 7(11): 550.

Elman M., Frank I., Cohen-Froman H., Harth Y. Effective treatment of atrophic and icepick acne scars using deep non-ablative radiofrequency and multisource fractional RF skin resurfacing. J Cosmet Dermatol 2012; 2: 267–272.

Esler W.P., Tesz G.J., Hellerstein M.K. et al. Human sebum requires de novo lipogenesis, which is increased in acne vulgaris and suppressed by acetyl-CoA carboxylase inhibition. Sci Transl Med 2019; 11(492): 8465.

Fabbrocini G., Annunziata M.C., D'Arco V. et al. Acne scars: pathogenesis, classification and treatment. Dermatol Res Pract 2010; 2010: 893080.

Fabbrocini G., Fardella N., Monfrecola A. et al. Acne scarring treatment using skin needling. Clin Exp Dermatol 2009; 34: 874–879.

Fritsch M., Orfanos C.E., Zouboulis C.C. Sebocytes are the key regulators of androgen homeostasis in human skin. J Invest Dermatol 2001; 116(5): 793–800.

Garg V.K., Sinha S., Sarkar R. Glycolic acid peels versus salicylic–mandelic acid peels in active acne vulgaris and postacne scarring and hyper-pigmentation: a comparative study. Dermatol Surg 2009; 35: 59–65.

Gelfond M.L., Panova O.S., Slovkhodov E.K., Zhukoff O.V. Photodynamic therapy in oncodermatology and cosmetology. Apparatnaya Cosmetologia 2017; 2: 36–44.

Goodarzi A., Mozafarpoor S., Bodaghabadi M., Mohamadi M. The potential of probiotics for treating acne vulgaris: a review of literature on acne and microbiota. Dermatol Ther 2020; 33(3): 13279.

Goodman G.J., Baron J.A. Postacne scarring: a qualitative global scarring grading system. Dermatol Surg 2006; 32: 1458–1466.

Greenhalch T. Fundamentals of evidence-based medicine. Translated from English, edited by I.N. Denisov and K.I. Saitkulov. GEOTAR-Media, 2009.

Harth Y., Elman M., Ackerman E., Frank I. Depressed acne scars — effective, minimal downtime treatment with a novel smooth motion non-insulated microneedle radio-frequency technology. J Cosmet Dermatol 2014; 4: 212–218.

Hellman J. Long term follow-up results of a fractional radio frequency ablative treatment of acne vulgaris and related acne scars. J Cosmet Dermatol Sci App 2016; 6: 100–104.

Hellman J., Yao J. Novel histological evidence of collagen and elastin regeneration in fractional RF-treated acne scars. J Cosmet Dermatol Sci App 2019; 9: 155–164.

Inoue T., Miki Y., Kakuo S. et al. Expression of steroidogenic enzymes in human sebaceous glands. J Endocrinol 2014; 222(3): 301–312.

Jacob C.I., Dover J.S., Kaminer M.S. Acne scarring: a classification system and review of treatment options. J Am Acad Dermatol. 2001; 45(1): 109–117.

Jarrousse V., Castex-Rizz N., Khammar A., Dreno B. Zinc salts inhibit in vitro Toll-like receptor 2 surface expression by keratinocytes. Eur J Dermatol 2007; 17(6): 492–496.

Joseph J.H., Shamban A., Eaton L. et al. Polymethylmethacrylate collagen gel-injectable dermal filler for full face atrophic acne scar correction. Dermatol Surg 2019; 45(12): 1558–1566.

Jung Y.R., Hwang C., Ha J.M. et al. Hyaluronic acid decreases lipid synthesis in sebaceous glands. J Invest Dermatol 2017; 137(6): 1215–1222.

Jung Y.R., Kim S.J., Sohn K.C. et al. Regulation of lipid production by light-emitting diodes in human sebocytes. Arch Dermatol Res 2015; 307(3): 265–273.

Kanazawa N. Designation of autoinflammatory skin manifestations with specific genetic backgrounds. Front Immunol 2020; 11: 475.

Katz B. The fate of active acne and acne scars following treatment with fractional radiofrequency. J Drugs Dermatol 2019; 18(12): 217–221.

Kircik L.H. Advances in the understanding of the pathogenesis of inflammatory acne. J Drugs Dermatol 2016; 15 (Suppl 1): 7–10.

Kircik L.H. Why do we need another moisturizer for our acne patients? J Drugs Dermatol 2014; 13(8): 88.

Kircik L.H. Importance of vehicles in acne therapy. J Drugs Dermatol 2011; 10(6): 17–S23.

Knackstedt R., Knackstedt T., Gatherwright J. The role of topical probiotics in skin conditions: a systematic review of animal and human studies and implications for future therapies. Exp Dermatol 2020; 29(1): 15–21.

Koike S., Akaishi S., Nagashima Y. et al. Nd:YAG laser treatment for keloids and hypertrophic scars: An analysis of 102 cases. PRS Global Open 2014; 2(12): 272.

Koren A., Isman G., Cohen S. et al. Efficacy of a combination of diluted calcium hydroxylapatite-based filler and an energy-based device for the treatment of facial atrophic acne scars. Clin Exp Dermatol 2019; 44(5): 171–176.

Korneeva R.V. Perfluorine compounds in injectable cosmetology: a new approach to the correction of aesthetic problems. Injection Methods in Cosmetology 2018; 4: 66–74.

Korneeva R.V. PFC Oxy®: a new embodiment of "blue blood" properties. Cosmetics and Medicine 2019; 4: 34.

Kravvas G., Al-Niaimi F. a systematic review of treatments for acne scarring. Part 1: Non-energy-based techniques. Scars, Burns & Healing 2017; 3: 2059513117695312.

Lee S.J., Seok J., Jeong S.Y. et al. Facial pores: Definition, causes, and treatment options. Dermatol Surg 2016; 42(3): 277–285.

Li W.H., Fassih A., Binner C. et al. Low-level red LED light inhibits hyperkeratinization and inflammation induced by unsaturated fatty acid in an in vitro model mimicking acne. Lasers Surg Med 2018; 50(2): 158–165.

Li Z.J., Park S.B., Sohn K.C. et al. Regulation of lipid production by acetylcholine signalling in human sebaceous glands. J Dermatol Sci 2013; 72(2): 116–122.

Lichtenberger R., Simpson M.A., Smith C. et al. Genetic architecture of acne vulgaris. J Eur Acad Dermatol Venereol 2017; 31(12): 1978–1990.

McCoy W.H., Otchere E., Rosa B.A. et al. Skin ecology during sebaceous drought — How skin microbes respond to isotretinoin. J Invest Dermatol 2018; 139(3): 732–735.

Mirnezami M., Rahimi H. Is oral omega-3 effective in reducing mucocutaneous side effects of isotretinoin in patients with acne vulgaris? Dermatol Res Pract 2018; 2018: 6974045.

Nast A., Eming S., Fluhr J. et al. German S2k guidelines for the therapy of pathological scars (hypertrophic scars and keloids). J Dtsch Dermatol Ges 2012; 10(10): 747–762.

Nettis E., Colanardi M.C., Ferrannini A., Tursi A. Antihistamines as important tools for regulating inflammation. Curr Med Chem — Anti-Inflamm Anti-Allergy Agents 2005; 4: 81–89.

Nikolaeva N.N. Ineffectiveness of external therapy in patients with acne: Current solutions. Cosmetics and Medicine 2019; 1: 8–13.

Pelle E., McCarthy J., Seltmann H. et al. Identification of histamine receptors and reduction of squalene levels by an antihistamine in sebocytes. J Invest Dermatol 2008; 128(5): 1280–1285.

Poetschke J., Gerd G. Current options for the treatment of pathological scarring. J Dtsch Dermatol Ges 2016; 14(5): 467–478.

Pondeljak N., Lugović-Mihić L. Stress-induced interaction of skin immune cells, hormones, and neurotransmitters. Clin Ther 2020; 42(5): 757–770.

Rahanskaya E.M. Pigmentary disorders: a review of the possibilities of hardware cosmetology. Hardware Cosmetology 2016; 3: 6–19.

Rivera A.E. Acne scarring: a review and current treatment modalities. J Am Acad Dermatol 2008; 59(4): 659–676.

Rocha M.A., Bagatin E. Skin barrier and microbiome in acne. Arch Dermatol Res 2018; 310(3): 181–185.

Roh M.R., Chung H.J., Chung K.Y. Effects of various parameters of the 1064 nm Nd:YAG laser for the treatment of enlarged facial pores. J Dermatolog Treat 2009; 20: 223–228.

Rubin M.G., Kim K., Logan A.C. Acne vulgaris, mental health and omega-3 fatty acids: a report of cases. Lipids Health Dis 2008; 7: 36.

Sachdeva S. Lactic acid peeling in superficial acne scarring in Indian skin. J Cosmet Dermatol 2010; 9: 246–248.

Sage R.J., Lopiccolo M.C., Liu A. et al. Subcuticular incision versus naturally sourced porcine collagen filler for acne scars: a randomized split-face comparison. Dermatol Surg 2011; 37: 426–431.

Sapra S., Stewart J.A., Mraud K. et al. a Canadian study of the use of poly-L-lactic acid dermal implant for the treatment of hill and valley acne scarring. Dermatol Surg 2015; 41: 587–594.

Saunte D.M.L., Gaitanis G., Hay R.J. Malassezia-associated skin diseases, the use of diagnostics and treatment. Front Cell Infect Microbiol 2020; 10: 112.

Sekhon A.K., Zergham A.S., Tserenpil G. et al. The association between polycystic ovary syndrome and its dermatological manifestations. Review. Cureus 2020; 12(2): 6855.

Sharad J. Combination of microneedling and glycolic acid peels for the treatment of acne scars in dark skin. J Cosmet Dermatol 2011; 10: 317–323.

Spring L.K., Krakowski A.C., Alam M. et al. Isotretinoin and timing of procedural interventions: a systematic review with consensus recommendations. JAMA Dermatol 2017; 153: 802–809.

Takagi Y., Ning X., Takahashi A. et al. The efficacy of a pseudo-ceramide and eucalyptus extract containing lotion on dry scalp skin. Clin Cosmet Investig Dermatol 2018; 11: 141–148.

Tan J.K.L., Stein Gold L.F., Alexis A.F. et al. Current concepts in acne pathogenesis: Pathways to inflammation. Semin Cutan Med Surg 2018; 37(3S): 60–62.

Taub A.F., Garretson C.B. Treatment of acne scars of skin types II to V by sublative fractional bipolar radiofrequency and bipolar radiofrequency combined with diode laser. J Cosmet Dermatol 2011; 4: 18–27.

Urakova D.S., Kalashnikova N.G. Spatially modulated ablation (SMA) in the correction of striae. Hardware Cosmetology 2015; 3: 58–62.

Volkova N.V., Glazkova L.K., Khomchenko V.V., Sadick N.S. Novel method for facial rejuvenation using Er:YAG laser equipped with a spatially modulated ablation module: An open prospective uncontrolled cohort study. J Cosmet Laser Ther 2017; 19(1): 25–29.

Waldman A., Bolotin D., Arndt K.A. et al. ASDS guidelines task force: Consensus recommendations regarding the safety of lasers, dermabrasion, chemical peels, energy devices, and skin surgery during and after isotretinoin use. Dermatol Surg 2017; 43: 1249–1262.

Wang D., Duncan B., Li X., Shi J. The role of NLRP3 inflammasome in infection-related, immune-mediated and autoimmune skin diseases. J Dermatol Sci 2020; 98(3): 146–151.

Whang S.W., Lee S.E., Kim J.M. et al. Effects of α-melanocyte-stimulating hormone on calcium concentration in SZ95 sebocytes. Exp Dermatol 2011; 20(1): 19–23.

Wollina U., Goldman A. Fillers for the improvement in acne scars. Clin Cosmet Investig Dermatol 2015; 8: 493–499.

Xia J., Hu G., Hu D. et al. Concomitant use of 1,550-nm nonablative fractional laser with low-dose isotretinoin for the treatment of acne vulgaris in Asian patients: a randomized split-face controlled study. Dermatol Surg 2018; 44(9): 1201–1208.

Yu Y., Dunaway S., Champer J. et al. Changing our microbiome: Probiotics in dermatology. Br J Dermatol. 2020; 182(1): 39–46.

Zachariae H. Delayed wound healing and keloid formation following argon laser treatment or dermabrasion during isotretinoin treatment. Br J Dermatol 1988; 118: 703–706.

Zhang L., Anthonavage M., Huang Q. et al. Proopiomelanocortin peptides and sebogenesis. Ann N Y Acad Sci 2003; 994: 154–161.

Zhou M., Gan Y., He C. et al. Lipidomics reveals skin surface lipid abnormity in acne in young men. Br J Dermatol 2018; 179(3): 732–740.

Zhou M., Wang H., Yang M. et al. Lipidomic analysis of facial skin surface lipids reveals an altered lipid profile in infant acne. Br J Dermatol 2020; 182(3): 817–818.

Zhou M., Xie H., Cheng L., Li J. Clinical characteristics and epidermal barrier function of papulopustular rosacea: a comparison study with acne vulgaris. Pak J Med Sci 2016; 32(6): 1344–1348.

www.ingramcontent.com/pod-product-compliance
Lightning Source LLC
Chambersburg PA
CBHW052021030426

42335CB00026B/3236